Also by N.D. London

My Healing Plan:
The ultimate journal to help you to embark on your healing journey.

Affirmations: 33 affirmations that will transform your life.
How to manifest all that you want, wish and desire.

Anxious about being anxious:
Simple techniques to calm the mind.

www.ndlondon.co.uk
www.divine-distribution.co.uk

cancersupportnet
nd.london
myhealingplan

Cancer

Diagnosis

What you are NOT told

Coping with a cancer diagnosis
and never giving up hope

N.D. London

Copyright

Disclaimer

This book details the author's personal experiences with, and opinions about cancer. The author is not medically trained and is by no means a healthcare provider or professional.

The author is providing this book and its contents on an "as is" basis and makes no representations or warranties of any kind with respect to this book or its contents. The statements made are not intended to diagnose, treat, cure, or prevent any condition or disease and does not claim to provide all information on the treatments or tests available for cancer sufferers. If you or your loved one has been diagnosed with cancer or you have concerns about your health, you should always seek professional advice.

Please ensure that you consult with your own physician or healthcare specialist regarding any suggestions and recommendations made in this book.

The author of this book will not be held liable for damages arising out of, or in connection with, the use of this book. The author is not prescribing any medicine or supplements and, by reading this book, you are accepting that any action taken after reading this book is done so at your own risk.

This is a comprehensive limitation of liability that applies to all damages of any kind, including (without limitation) compensatory; direct, indirect, or consequential damages; loss of data, income, or profit; loss of, or damage to, property; and claims of third parties.

You understand that this book is not intended as a substitute for consultation with a licensed healthcare practitioner, such as yours or your loved one's oncologist, physician, or general practitioner. Before you or your loved one begin any healthcare program, or makes lifestyle changes in any way, you should consult your physician or another licensed healthcare practitioner to ensure that you are in good health and that the examples contained in this book will not harm you.

Contents

Acknowledgements

I would like to say a huge thank you to my wonderful mum for being herself and being the best parent anyone could ask for. Your strength, beauty and heart, especially at this time in your life is admirable and we are honoured to be your children. Thank you to my stepfather for trying his best in this caregiving role that has been sent his way and for taking care of my mum. Thank you to my husband Dean and my beautiful girls, Sienna and Nyah, for being my world and keeping me motivated to write this book so that I can hopefully help others.

Thank you to my sister for being so wonderful and a huge part of our support network. Thank you to Ariya and Eden for keeping Nanny smiling alongside your cousins, and thank you to my auntie for always being there with treatment ideas and inspiration while providing my mum with all of the support that she could ever need from a sister.

Thank you to my friends and soul sisters; Joanie for sharing her own treatment stories and ideas, and Keisha for the love and continuous sounding board that you are.

Thank you to all of my mum's friends that have helped her on this journey.

Thank you to the amazing doctors, oncologists, healthcare practitioners, herbalists, and healers that have shared their research and advice with me. I am truly humbled and grateful for the amount of help and assistance that I have received.

A huge thank you to everyone for their love and support shown during this time and process.

****

Introduction

'Your body is your temple.' How many times have we heard that and just brushed it to one side? 'Health is wealth' is another great one that gets thrown around by so many, but how many of us process the words and take them literally? It's only when we are hit with the devastating news that our body is not functioning as it should be, or that we or someone we love is riddled with some kind of illness or disease that we appreciate and long for the health that was once there. It is only when we are faced with something like disease or death that we learn to appreciate how much we want health and life! It's funny how the human mind works, isn't it?

Next time we hear these phrases, we should stop to acknowledge them as never were truer words uttered; health most definitely is wealth, as without it we truly suffer.

In this book, you will accompany me on the journey of when my mum discovered that she had cancer. We will look into how this devastating disease has affected our whole family and made us better people because of it. You will read along to discover some of the revolutionary treatments that are available for cancer sufferers, whether used to supplement conventional treatment methods or used as standalone therapies. This book has been designed as a resource guide that can help you to open your mind to the various options available, which will hopefully help you or your loved one to heal, as you can only make the right options if you are fully informed and aware of what's out there. While reading the chapters of this book, you will encounter stories of survivorship wrapped in words of kindness and compassion that will help you to persevere on your journey of hope and healing, whether for yourself or for a loved one.

I am not a doctor or medical professional, but what I am is the daughter of a stage 4 cancer sufferer who has tried my absolute best to research and look into all of the available options accessible to us in order to help my mum on her journey of healing.

This book is a great place to start if you or someone that you love is coming to terms with a cancer diagnosis, as I have aimed to make the information contained as easy to read and digestible as possible.

****

Chapter One

Understanding The Diagnosis And The Difference Between Cure, Remission, And Elongating Life

Hearing that someone has cancer has become a casual thing for most of us. We hear and see it everywhere: in films, on social media, and on the news. It is so common in this day and age that we have become desensitised to this heart-breaking and destructive disease. That is, of course, until you are diagnosed with it or someone we love tells us that they have it. Once it sinks in, we come to the realisation that we could be in danger of losing so much to this humongous disease, and that's when we start researching and looking for a cure.

If you are like me, you will go out there and look at all the possible and impossible alternatives available. I am here to tell you that like you, I believe that there is hope for cancer sufferers, and in this book I aim to show you some of the different things that you can try and test on your journey.

Prior to delving deeper into the alternative treatment options available, I think that it's important for you to understand the initial staging and grading process that doctors have used in order to reach their diagnosis.

Diagnosis Staging And Grading

In order to properly assess the disease and its progression, doctors have a system in place where they put the cancer found into stages and grades in order to understand what they are dealing with.

There are five stages:

» **Stage 0** – indicates that the cancer is in the same place it started and hasn't spread.

» **Stage I** – the cancer looks small and has not spread yet.
» **Stage II** – the cancer has grown a bit but hasn't spread anywhere else yet.
» **Stage III** - the cancer is bigger and has possibly spread to the surrounding lymph nodes and/or tissues.
» **Stage IV** – the cancer has spread from its initial place to at least one other organ, also known as metastatic cancer.

A grading system is also used to categorise the way the cancer looks under a microscope and how fast it is growing.

There are three grades:
» **Grade I** - cancer cells that look similar to normal cells and aren't growing quickly.
» **Grade II** - cancer cells that don't look like normal cells and are growing faster than normal cells.
» **Grade III** - cancer cells that look abnormal and are growing and spreading more aggressively.

After allocating the cancer a certain stage and grade, the doctor will then advise the patient of the treatment option or options that are available to them. Once we have this information from the doctors and we begin our own research into the treatment options available, the two terms you will see more often than not are 'cure' and 'remission'. It is important to understand the difference between the two in order to correctly assess what steps to take next.

Cure And Remission

First, remission can be of two types: partial and complete.

When a patient is first diagnosed, various tests would have to be done in order to assess the exact stage and extent of their cancer. The most common tests done are blood tests, biopsies, CT scans, PET scans, or MRI.

Once the doctor has assessed the exact stage of cancer, they will recommend starting a therapy. This therapy will usually include a combination of surgery, chemotherapy, radiation, hormone therapy, immunotherapy, or biologic therapy.

After starting the therapy, and after a certain period of time, the patient will be assessed in order to check how the disease is responding. The disease will then be classified as either progressing, responding to treatment, or stable. For patients whose disease is responding to treatment, the doctor would usually use the term 'remission'. Sometimes it will be 'partial remission' and other times it will be 'complete remission'. The term 'remission' itself means that the cancer is improving measurably. As we mentioned before, remission can be either partial or complete.

Partial remission is referred to when a patient partly responds to therapy, either showing clinical improvement or a radiographic one. However, in partial remission, there is still clear evidence of the disease remaking in the organism. The disease is improving overall, but it is still present. Partial remission can also be mixed, where the therapy removed some of the tumours, or one and left some intact, or only affected them partly. Sometimes, partially remittent patients can take a break from the treatment as long as their cancer doesn't start spreading again and is being controlled.

In some cases, complete remission has been experienced by patients. This occurs when there is no evidence of cancer left in the body by any means or tests available. This term is often used when the patient finishes the whole treatment and tests come back negative. In a breast cancer patient, for example, after a successful excision of the breast, the patient is technically in complete remission. The doctors will not refer to it like that until all of the follow-up tests have been completed and all results reflect that there is no longer any cancer cells visible.

After understanding the term 'remission' and how it is used, it is also important to compare the terms 'remission' and 'cure'. Contrary to what it sounds like, complete remission is not synonymous with being cured. In complete remission, there is evidence that cancer is not present at a certain point in time, however, there can still be a risk of it coming back.

If you remain in remission for 5 years or more, some doctors and physicians may declare the patient as 'cured' as there is now no evidence of the cancer in the body and there is a low chance of it returning. There are, however, some cancers where no known timespan can indicate whether or not the patient will ever be truly cured or if they will have a longer complete remission.

There are also cases in the last stage of cancer when the cancer has spread too widely and is not responding to treatment any more. This is when modern medicine has no cure. The doctors will then approximate the amount of time the patient has until the cancer gets to the vital organs and stops them from working. In this case, a patient can be in different scenarios. If the cancer still responds to treatment in a minimalistic way, then it is possible for their life to be elongated. With this in mind, the patient will have the option to go through an aggressive treatment (because at this stage the cancer is also aggressive) for the hope of gaining some more years or even months, or to stop the treatment completely and to make peace with the outcome.

In modern medicine, this seems to be recurring more often than not, which can look pretty hopeless objectively. However, if you look at the human body through thicker lenses, other options will become apparent.

There are various alternative therapies available now that have been proven to increase a cancer patient's chance of survival, even when conventional doctors have given the patient an end of life prognosis.

****

Chapter Two

My Story: Hearing
My Mother's Diagnosis And Prognosis Shock

It was a dreary rainy December day in London. My sister and I were sitting at my dining room table, drumming our fingers, waiting for our mum and our stepfather to arrive. They had been to the hospital to get the results back from an MRI scan that my mum had had, as a previous x-ray had shown a mass in her left lung. We were praying for it to be something else but deep down, in a place that we didn't want to admit, we already knew what the outcome was. We had discussed the possibility of all eventualities, had Googled the hell out of 'lung mass', and we knew all of the symptoms for the various lung conditions that it could have been, but the gut never lies.

When my mum and our stepfather arrived at my house after the appointment, the look on their faces told the story. They sat down and unwaveringly stated that the MRI had shown that our wonderful mum had stage 4 lung cancer. It was a conversation that I've replayed a million times over, looking for any emotion to show on my mum's face, but she was blank as always as she was more concerned about what we were feeling rather than how she felt! As she dealt us this devastating blow, she was calmly saying that the mass on her lung had spread to her lymph nodes, collar, and her right lung. Her oncologist had informed her that she had terminal stage 4 (NSCLC) non-small cell lung cancer.

My mum had not been given a prognosis yet but due to the constant research I had been doing over the past weeks, I was aware that the prognosis was not good for stage 4 lung cancer. In tune with my optimistic personality, I started on the positive words that I could share with them all around the table, saying how we need to get a second opinion (that you should always get) and how we can look at all of the alternative treatments available. However, while I was saying these words, my head was hurting and my heart was breaking.

Coming To Terms With The Diagnosis

The weeks following this awful news were spent reading numerous books on cancer and researching the specific cancer that my mum had been diagnosed with; (NSCLC) non-small cell lung cancer. I watched all of the documentaries that I could find and I tried to equip myself with as much knowledge as possible in order to understand the disease and the symptoms associated with it. I am incredibly close to my mum and when I received the news, my anxiety hit the roof! I decided then and there that my role would be to research, research, research. This is when I started my journey of looking into everything that could hopefully cure her or, at the very least, elongate her life.

The first piece of advice is to always get a second opinion. Sometimes it's easy to forget that doctors are still human and humans can make mistakes; it's always best to find another doctor who has a specialty in the particular cancer that you or your loved one has in order to provide a second opinion, as every cancer patient is entitled to one.

While You Are Waiting

Due to my mum being a UK NHS patient, there was a period of waiting between receiving her diagnosis, having a biopsy taken, and receiving her first appointment with an oncologist (a doctor that specialises in cancer). During this interim phase, prior to her first appointment with an oncologist, we had started to research cancer and diet, and come to the conclusion that a plant-based, organic, alkaline diet would be the best and easiest thing that could be implemented immediately in order to kick-start her healing journey.

The logic behind this is that my mum would be flooding her body with all of the required nutrients, vitamins, and minerals, which would theoretically help her body to be as strong as it could be. This was all done in order to prepare her body and help her to be in the best possible condition ahead of starting any cancer treatment.

First Appointment

For my mum's first oncology appointment, we all went along to try and gain an understanding of my mum's situation. We were armed with a huge list of questions that we had composed in preparation. I have listed some of the questions below for your information as they may come in handy if you are having to go through this:

Questions For The Oncologist

1. *What is the exact diagnosis? Is it the type of cancer that spreads quickly? If so, has it spread and where has it spread to?*

2. *For what purpose would any treatment be? Would it be curative or palliative, i.e. to extend life, cure the cancer, or is it to create a better quality of life until the end?*

3. *Have you, or will you be carrying out any targeted therapies such as metabolic testing or chemosensitivity testing?*

4. *What are the treatment options available? (Ask for a breakdown of each option with the names of the drugs that will be taken).*

5. *What are the side effects and the purpose of each treatment?*

6. *Have you taken these drugs yourself? Would you take them or would you prescribe them to a close family member if they were diagnosed with this form of cancer?*

7. *How old are the drugs being recommended?*

8. *Is Targeted Low Dose Insulin Potentiation Therapy (TLD/IPT) an option that they would offer? (This is chemo with insulin. It is a targeted therapy and is 1/10 the strength of normal chemo. This is a good alternative option to full-blown chemo, as it will not target normal healthy cells).*

9. How many treatment cycles are there for each treatment option? How long do you expect the treatment cycles to last for, and how long is each treatment session (if chemo or radiotherapy)?
10. How do you advise the patient and us as a family to prepare for treatment?
11. What are the 2-year and 5-year survival rates for this type of cancer, and is there a research paper available with the breakdown of the participant's age and health status, alongside their type of cancer available to us?
12. If the patient was to refuse the conventional treatments offered, what would the prognosis be?
13. If successfully treated, what are the chances of the cancer coming back?
14. What do they think caused the cancer? Is it genetic?
15. Would you recommend any dietary and lifestyle changes?
16. Would you recommend any supplements and/or alternative treatments?
17. How many people do you personally know in your clinic that have been cured or survived with a good quality of life beyond 5 or 10 years?
18. If you decide not to do chemo, can you still have the oncologist's support for regular blood tests and scans?

***Try to get a printed copy of all of your test results
and diagnosis for your own reference***

My mum's oncologist had clearly missed the module of bedside manner at medical school, as all of our questions were ignored. She was one of those doctors that was offended that we dare ask her any questions.

When we asked the oncologist about any dietary advice that she would give, she suggested carrying on as normal, eating as she had been, with the option of even having a glass of wine in the evening!

The advice from all doctors, I feel, should be for them to tell all patients to try to be as healthy as possible in order to prepare the body for the battle ahead – as it is a battle and no matter what you have been told, there is still a chance that you can fight it, cure it, or outlive your prognosis by years!!

The doctor proceeded to advise my mum to 'get her affairs in order.' She then informed us that the results from the first biopsy taken of the tumour had come back inconclusive (as the doctors did not take enough cells to sample). This sample should have provided my mum with details of the specific mutation of NSCLC that she had, as this would therefore determine any specific treatment options available. As you can imagine, not having the biopsy results dealt another blow to my mum as it would mean she would need to be booked in for another biopsy and would then need to wait at least another month for the new results. This only added to the stress levels.

During the time waiting for the results of the second biopsy, I managed to research and secure an appointment with a doctor who dealt specifically with the ablation technique and the use of it on lung cancer patients. Initially, the consultation started off well with him looking at the scans, images, etc. and discussing the ablation technique but, as soon as he realised that the cancer was so far spread, our initial positivity was shattered by the confirmation that the cancer really was too advanced and the option of a targeted therapy drug or full-blown chemo would be the only options available for her from the doctors at this point.

At this time, my mum was unsure if she even wanted to undergo chemotherapy due to the side effects associated with it. We had also read that several oncologists, when personally asked if they would undergo chemotherapy themselves, had said that they would decline it. My mum was left considering what she would do if chemo was her only available option.

During this whole time period, I was gaining knowledge of the various treatments available and was discussing my findings with her and my auntie who was also doing non-stop research.

My mum, through this, was very trusting and was 'up' for trying most things that we were suggesting. So, here begins our journey into the alternative therapies that are on offer.

12

As I had been on a 'research rampage', I was equipped with all kinds of information. What follows are details of some treatment options that we have explored that may prove revolutionary in yours or your loved one's cancer journey.

In this book, at the end of each chapter I outline my mum's own experience with some of the treatments mentioned. I hope her story will inspire you to have hope and not give up!

****

Chapter Three

Conventional Therapies: Chemo,

Immunotherapy, And Radiation

Even though this book has been primarily designed to help people to find alternative treatments for cancer, it has to be noted that conventional methods can be effective for a lot of people. It is often recommended that people first try conventional means of healing cancer if they are in the physical state to do so. Many of these have harmful side effects and can seriously decrease your quality of life, however, when your life is on the line it may be worth looking into these treatments.

You do not have to go into it blindly. I have tried to compose and simplify most of the important information regarding these treatments so that you or your loved one can feel prepared.

Chemotherapy

Let's start with the type of treatment that you may be most familiar with: chemotherapy. Chemotherapy alludes to drugs that are generally used to treat cancer in patients. Chemotherapy drugs work fundamentally by assaulting the rapidly separating cells. By interfering with some of the fundamental mechanisms that drive cell division, they cause the cell to decay and die. While there are numerous chemo agents on the market today, it is best that we focus on three of the most common types of chemotherapy and their derived drugs: alkylating agents, anti-metabolites, and plant alkaloids. Each class harms cells in an unexpected way.

Alkylating agents work by joining to the DNA helix and keeping DNA from uncoiling. This impairs DNA replication which means that the cell can't divide and multiply. Typical examples of these medications are cyclophosphamide, chlorambucil, and nitrogen mustard. Alkylating agents are usually utilised to treat lymphomas, leukemias, breast, prostate, and other types of cancer.

Anti-metabolites are drugs that interfere with DNA production. As cancer cells divide more rapidly than non-cancerous cells, the anti-metabolytes will affect cancer cell replication by inhibiting cell division, causing cancer cell death. For instance, 5 fluorouracil, or 5FU, is a type of treatment that keeps cells from making the DNA building blocks called thymine, which is essential for the proper functioning of cells when it comes to their survival.

Plant alkaloids are chemotherapy sedatives that keep cells from collecting microtubules. Microtubules are fibre-like structures that pull the arrangement of chromosomes into every daughter cell during division. Without microtubules, cell division can not be completed and the cell dies. Examples of plant alkaloid medications incorporate vinblastine and vincristine. A patient's illness will for the most part adapt to one type of chemotherapy and become immune to it over time. This is why the vast majority of medical practitioners that focus on treating cancer will combine multiple types of chemotherapy in order to keep it from adapting and surviving.

Targeted Low Dose Insulin Potentiation Therapy

What a lot of doctors will not tell you is that there is a chemotherapy available in lower doses which is given at a tenth of the strength of conventional chemotherapy. This form of low dose chemo is called Targeted Low Dose Insulin Potentiation Therapy (TLD/IPT) and is given to patients on a more regular basis over a longer period of time. This therapy has been proven to have the same effect as full-blown chemo in several trials that have been conducted.

The benefit of low dose chemo is that, as the level of toxic drugs pumped into the body is much lower than what is given in conventional chemo, the healthy cells are not all bombarded at the same time and killed along with the cancer cells (which allows some of the immune system to stay intact). Low dose chemo may also stop the growth of new blood vessels that tumours reqire to grow.

Conventional chemo is not targeted and is usually prescribed in doses that are so strong it will kill off the majority of your healthy cells, damaging your immune system along with killing the cancer cells. The low dose chemo will leave you or your loved one, with less side effects than if treated with conventional chemo.

Unfortunately, at this time, low dose chemo is only available privately in the UK, but there are several clinics that offer this treatment. If you are elsewhere in the world and have private healthcare, your treatment may be covered in your insurance plan, so it is worth investigating.

Chemo Or Cold Caps

If you or someone you love is about to embark on the journey of chemotherapy and are worried about side effects such as hair loss, there is something called a chemo or a cold cap that is available for chemotherapy patients for a charge. These caps are applied to the scalp/hair and effectively freeze hair follicles so that the chemotherapy agents are unable to attack the hair which will lead to hair loss. The downside to these caps is that some patients have reported that they are very uncomfortable and heavy to wear. They also give some patients headaches and require an extra 1.5 hours on average before each treatment and 1.5 hours after each treatment to apply and remove.

Immunotherapy

Our body is equipped with cells that act as an aggressive swarm, which helps our system to defend itself and fight foreign invaders. These are known as immune cells. Some of these immune cells are called T cells and B cells, and are programmed to get rid of foreign invaders like viruses and bacteria. T cells release toxins against the intruders and B cells make antibodies to neutralise them. It has been known for quite a while that immune cells can recognise cancer cells as foreign invaders and attack them by secreting special biological weapons.

T cells continuously scan the surface of cells through the T cell receptor, or TCR. The TCR works as a barcode scanning machine and the peptides presented on the cells are unique barcodes that help the T cell to identify it. This function of the T cells is called surveillance. If T cells recognise these peptides as normal then the T cells move on, but if the peptides come from foreign invader proteins then the T cells get activated to attack the invader cell with the aforementioned biological weapons to eliminate the intruder. T cells secrete certain chemicals called cytokines, and these molecules punch holes into the cells that contain the invading organisms, thus killing them.

Abnormal peptides, like those that are created when cancerous proteins break down, are recognised by the TCR as foreign. This then activates the T cells to kill the cancer cells. But if the immune system can recognise and eliminate cancer, then why do people develop cancer? The simple answer is that sometimes the immune system fails to do its job. The immune response against cancer may not be strong enough to fully deal with the scale of invasion, as it was never designed to do so. It may even be that the cancer cells have managed to evade the immune system.

The problem with cancer is that it is complex in nature and intelligent. Tumours, or a group of cancer cells, can build a defence network against our immune system. These defence mechanisms can either prevent the immune army from entering the tumour, or inhibit the T cells from functioning properly. For example, tumours can express attack molecules on their surface that bind to the T cells and inhibit their killing activity; these molecules are called checkpoints, and examples are PD 1 and CTLA 4. The tumour can also secrete protein factors and cytokines that inhibit T cells from attacking and killing cancer cells, and can also turn the T cells into biological friends of the tumour. The story gets even worse, because the now cancer-obedient T cells can then deactivate other T cells, thus rendering them useless in the fight against cancer.

Immunotherapy boosts and stimulates certain parts of a persons own immune system which enables it to work in a harder and smarter way to find, attack and destroy cancer cells. Immunotherapy is one of the most important recent revolutions in the history of cancer treatment. Your doctor will usually investigate if it can be used as a method in your treatment plan.

Please note that if you or your loved one is fighting cancer and has an existing autoimmune disease, immunotherapy may not be an option.

Radiation

Radiation is simply a spectrum of energy. We have exposure to radiation every day that comes from different sources. Radiation can be used in two different ways in terms of cancer treatment; it can have a curative intent or as a means of alleviating pain or other symptoms. This type of therapeutic radiation, when directed to a targeted area in the body, will cause damage to the DNA on a cellular level within cancer and that DNA damage translates to cell death. However, radiation can damage both cancer cells as well as normal tissues in the surrounding area.

Fortunately for your body, normal tissue can repair the damage caused to the DNA from radiotherapy much more effectively than cancer cells can, and therefore over time, the normal tissue is able to survive the radiation treatments that cause the targeted cancer cells to die.

Radiation is very personalised for each individual cancer patient and is based on the location of the tumour. There are multiple types of radiation therapy, one common method is known as external beam radiation therapy, which is administered by way of a machine. Another form of treatment is an internal treatment where radioactive material is placed inside the body to deliver the radiation to the cancerous cells. Each method has its drawbacks and benefits, but each has proven effective to help cancer patients in various circumstances.

Proton Beam Therapy

Proton beam therapy, or PBT, is a conventional method of radiation. This therapy uses a high energy beam of protons (light particles) to treat various forms of cancer. The benefit of this treatment is that it can directly target tumour cells due to its high level of precision. Various other radiation therapies available damage surrounding tissues, causing adverse side effects. For this reason, proton beam therapy is a great option for people who have cancer in sensitive areas, such as the spinal cord.

The procedure is usually considered painless and not many people experience any type of side effect from it. The NHS in the UK states that it is a reasonable approach for certain types of cancers and there are currently two centres in the country providing the therapy for free, dependent on your cancer type, with a third treatment centre being planned.

Yours or your loved one's oncologist may not offer this treatment as it may not be their preferred path for their patients. It is however, worth investigating if this therapy would work for yours or your loved one's specific cancer, as if it has shown positive results for similar cases, they may also have a case.

If you are not in the UK and radiation therapy has been suggested, it may be worth asking the oncologist if there is a proton beam therapy option available.

Making Decisions

You or your loved one may find it difficult at this time to make decisions due to all of the information that there is for you to process. You may find that everyone around you has an opinion on the path that you should take, but just remember that you always have a choice.

Sometimes alternative treatments alone can be enough to tackle certain cancers. In some cases it may be necessary to combine conventional treatments with alternative therapies in order to combat the cancer and strengthen the body, and sometimes conventional treatments such as chemo, even though it can often be stressful on the body, can help people to overcome a more advanced form of cancer.

The main thing to remember when making any decision, is that decisions should be made by the patient based on what feels right for them and according to their individual wants and needs. At this stage it would be appropriate to seek advice from an integrated or alternative cancer specialist as well as your doctors.

My Mother's Journey

Later on in my mum's cancer story, she was shown to have metastases in her brain, which is fairly common with the type of cancer that she has.

Previously she had non-cancerous brain tumours that were operated on 15 years prior to this, so we believe that the cancer may have been there upon initial diagnosis, but it may have been missed as there was some scar tissue present on the brain that the doctors may have mistaken as non-cancerous.

▶

One year after her initial diagnosis, when the brain metastases were spotted, my mum was prescribed 10 sessions of full-brain radiation over a 14-day period.

The side effects set in over 6 weeks after her final session and included weakness, lethargy, being sick, losing her hair, and burnt scalp and ears to name a few.*

*My aunt purchased a cream for my mum to help with the burns called Radiance skin care by Louise Brackenbury. It is a nourishing gel that can help to relieve the burning sensation and soreness caused by radiotherapy.

****

Chapter Four

Embracing Your Cancer,
Acceptance, And Cell Psychology

So you may be wondering how you can embrace something that is so destructive to yourself and the people around you, especially as cancer has so many elements to it that makes us so fearful; such as the thought of death and the worry of what happens to us or our loved ones beyond this life.

Fear is a natural state of being, however there are ways in which to turn this fear into something positive and let's face it, if you are faced with cancer or someone you love has been diagnosed, it makes no sense whatsoever to dwell on all of the possible negative outcomes. You need to be proactive and learn tactics to regress the cancer or elongate life, and you will need to do this by working with the cancer. This is when embracing the cancer comes into play.

Cancer has several stages that accompanies a diagnosis. These are recognised as denial, anger, bargaining, sadness and depression, and then acceptance. I would like you to focus on acceptance, as this can really help you or your loved one on this journey of healing.

I would like you to visualise your body as the amazing source of energy that it is; you are made up of trillions of cells and if cancer is present, it would usually only make up a small part of that. The cells that have invaded the body are causing havoc, yes, but when looking at the amount of cells that make up the body, the cancer is only taking over a small amount of these cells in comparison, so I would like you or your loved one to try to focus on that.

The cells affected may benefit from something that is called cell communication. It may sound 'out there' but many people have had great results on their healing journeys by placing themselves into a deep meditative state and embarking on cell communication. The theory is that as your cells are listening, you should talk to your body and all the cells, asking them what it is that you would like them to do. Tell them that you would like them to repair and fight off the cancer or unhealthy cells, let them know your desire for them to communicate with each other effectively and efficiently, in order for them to work together to provide you with a healthy body to live in. The words that you should use to communicate with your cells should be what sits right within your heart as the power to heal can come from many sources, but only if you have the faith and belief in the healing journey.

If you have been diagnosed with cancer, do not refer to yourself as a cancer sufferer. You are still you and it's advisable that you take some time to try to learn to separate yourself from the cancer objectively in order to evaluate your circumstance and make the best decisions and choices for your given scenario. Never feel rushed or pressured into making any decisions that you are unsure of or uncomfortable with. You now need to exert control, and your attitude needs to be shifted from negative to positive in order to not put your body through any more unnecessary stress, as emotional trauma can contribute to cancer growth.

You can then approach your healing with positivity and go into treatment with the mindset that your body has the power to heal from this. Tell your cells what you want them to do, allow them to hear you, and believe that this is what will occur. The link between mind and body is too vast to disregard. Never forget that human beings as a whole are complete living organisms and all of our cells communicate with each other in order for us to function.

Many cancer survivors have stated that a cancer diagnosis has given them the perspective and wisdom that they needed in order for them to analyse what truly makes them happy. This is a great example of how looking for the positive in every situation can take away

23

some of the negativity that is being experienced.

Making Plans

If you or someone you love is diagnosed with late-stage cancer, it's time to make plans. When I talk of making plans, I do not mean those of a funeral (although that does need to be covered and will be addressed in later chapters). What I mean is making plans to have as much fun as possible with the people you love. If it is a loved one that has been diagnosed, find out what they want to do and who they want to spend time with. Work with them to embrace the diagnosis as a kick-start to what they have been wanting to do. Encourage them to spend time with the people that matter, arrange that party or holiday that they want, albeit sooner than anticipated, write that list of what they want to achieve and get working through it.

Embrace your life and the people you love, see them through fresh eyes, appreciate what you have and the beauty of Earth, embrace everything; good and bad. When you are positive, you cause a shift in your mind and body. Suddenly, things that may have bothered you previously will now be seen as trivial and a waste of energy. Now is the time to embrace the beauty in everything, but not though sad eyes, through invigorated newly opened eyes, eyes that allow you to accept what is going on and will allow you to push through it anyway, as cancer or no cancer, we all have two things promised to us; that is life and death.

Rather than dwelling on all of the things that can and may go wrong, it's time to focus on what can and may go right, like you or your loved one potentially tackling cancer and living a life of healing, health and happiness.

Remember that all of us are different, our cells work differently from each other and therefore the outcomes of various situations will differ from person to person. This is why it's always wise to view a prognosis for what it is, an average for a random group of people. Your's or the body of your loved one may be similar to that person in the study who lived 2 or 20 years past the average prognosis stated, or the person whose cancer went into regression. You just do not know what will happen in your particular body until you try. So with this book in hand, it's time to look into the ways in which you can try to make a difference.

My Mother's Journey

I worked with my mum to create a list of things that she wanted to do and achieve while she was well enough, in order to remain positive. My mum's main aim was to spend as much time with her grandchildren as possible, as it is what makes her happy. We then set about making plans for different ways to do this.

We booked a big family holiday to make memories and have fun.

My sister and I arranged set days that my mum would come to our homes to spend time with us and the children. We kept positive by focusing on the immediate future!

My mum accepted her cancer and credits her faith for this. She was also able to embrace therapies with an open mind because of her faith in God and her healing journey.

****

Chapter Five

EMF, Bioresonance,

And Biomagnetism Therapy For Cancer

It is time that we start to delve deeper into various other alternative cancer treatments. Everything we have discussed thus far could be categorised as conventional. However, as you may well know, these things do not work for everyone. In fact, there are millions of people for whom they do not work for, therefore alternative treatments such as what follows may be required.

Rife Explained

The mainstream view of rife machines is that they are nothing but quackery, but there is no real surprise there as, quite often, any treatment that is alternative will likely be labelled as quackery. This is just an unfortunate side effect of living in a pharmaceutical-based system. So what exactly is a rife machine? Well in its most simple form, it is a frequency generator that's able to generate different frequencies and is able to control those frequencies with input signals.

The main idea behind this therapy is that cancer, as well as dangerous microorganisms, like to live in certain frequencies and if you send high-powered frequencies close to or at the frequency at which they operate then you can disrupt their internal functions. The first rife machine was invented by the American scientist known as Royal Raymond Rife (a name to remember). The frequencies that his machine produced were similar to, but not exactly the same as radio waves.

While he is known as the inventor of the rife machine, he expanded upon work previously conducted by Dr Albert Abrams. It was one of Abrams' fundamental views that diseases adhere to vibrational frequencies and that electrical pulses, such as the one from the rife machine, could kill them. The common name for this theory is radionics. In order to further solidify his belief, Rife developed a special type of microscope which he said was able to locate the electromagnetic frequency emitted from various cells (including bacteria, viruses, and cancer) by having different visual hues. Though many of his claims were not substantiated at the time, many anecdotal experiences would testify to the fact that his invention worked, saying that they have been able to beat everything from Lyme disease to cancer.

Unfortunately, there haven't been any large and controlled placebo-based studies which were then peer-reviewed in order to substantiate scientific backing for rife machines.

In the 1990's, many people started selling rife machines as part of a multi-level marketing business, a model that has garnered major scrutiny when it comes to its dubious business practices. This further diminished people's view of the treatment.

It is also a possibility that many within the conventional treatment community actively suppressed knowledge about successes using the rife treatment. One of the potential aggressors towards this treatment was the former American Medical Association leader Morris Fishbein, who was responsible for a lawsuit against Rife which ruined his career.

Despite some of the negativity surrounding rife machines, it is not impossible to ignore the anecdotal evidence that rife machines may indeed be a valuable treatment option for those looking to treat their cancer. The testimonials number in the thousands and as access to information about this treatment increases, so do the number of people positively affected by it. If you are considering treatment and would initially like to see how you get on with this type of treatment, there is currently a clinic offering rife therapy known as the Auror Scalar Technology clinic in Eindhoven, Netherlands, where you can go into the clinic and spend the day there taking in the frequencies that are emitted through the various rife machines placed around the centre. People benefit from regular sessions and some patients have moved near the clinic in order to regularly use the facilities. The clinic also offers various other therapies such as colloidal silver, gold, and indium treatment.

There are also several clinics worldwide that offer this therapy.

Risks

Mostly, rife machines are considered safe for individuals to undergo treatment with. The electrical pulses used are of a low enough frequency to not disrupt anything vital within your body. However, according to Cancer Research UK (2018), there have been instances where people have reported skin rashes and even low-level shocks. These instances are few and far between, and should not pose too much of an obstacle for anyone looking to pursue rife treatment.

Spooky 2

If you want to go ahead with purchasing a rife machine yourself, there are several available on the market; one being the Spooky 2 machine. It is an affordable option that you can buy for your own home and is portable enough to be carried to other locations without a problem. The Spooky 2 and other similar machines often come with all of the essential kit that you may require for starting your own rife therapy treatment and comes in various formats. In relation to the Spooky 2 machine; The XM model specialises in killing viruses and bacteria while the X model focuses on clearing toxins from the body. The latter is also far more powerful should you want to really commit to this treatment. Once again, please speak to your alternative health practitioner and oncologist before starting any new therapies that could interfere with your current treatment plan.

Biomagnetism

While not heavily promoted, biomagnetism is an emerging therapy in the energy treatment market that may be extremely beneficial for people fighting cancer.

Biomagnetism is a pioneering treatment that can correct imbalances within the body to increase people's wellbeing and health. Biomagnetic pair therapy uses magnets of opposing polarity in specific areas of the body to correct imbalances and restore a state of equilibrium and health. When areas of the body are in either an acidic or alkaline pH, the body's systems, most importantly the immune system, are unable to function adequately. These imbalances are a driving force behind many chronic illnesses. So by correcting the imbalances by using magnets, the cells, organs, and systems can function optimally to restore optimal health.

The practitioner will locate imbalances within the body by using a muscle testing technique and will then place magnets on the necessary areas. People have reported a vast number of benefits, including stress relief, increased immunity (which could be beneficial against cancer) and enhanced wellbeing. If you can repair bodily imbalances, your body will work more optimally, which can therefore affect how your body fights off the cancer.

There are several practitioners worldwide. Faye Coulson is a practitioner who is certified in Biomagnetism, Bioenergetics, and Biomagnetic Neuropsychology and is based in London, UK.

My Mother's Story

My mum received remote biomagnetism therapy where several imbalances were detected. My mum's therapist applied several different magnetic pairs to different areas of the body in order to create the correct set of magnetic frequencies that should be present in the body. She then provided the details of the various points that needed attention and supplied us with the details of the various magnets required for this in order for my mum to be able to treat herself between sessions.

****

Chapter Six

PRP For Cancer

Yours or your loved one's therapist may suggest pairing some therapies together that they believe can work in perfect harmony with each other in order to help achieve the freedom and healing that everyone is looking for. The next therapy had mixed reviews but, due to my mum's bleak prognosis, we decided that we would try this out anyway.

PRP Or Platelet-Rich-Plasma

PRP is usually obtained from blood. It is a by-product of using a method known as centrifugation on a blood sample which increases and concentrates platelet density within the blood, more specifically the plasma. The usual amount of platelets found after this process is conducted can be between three and fivefold the usual amount. The term 'platelet-rich-plasma' was first coined all the way back in the 1970s as a way of describing any plasma that had elevated levels of platelets when compared to a standard sample taken from the peripheries of the body.

After centrifugation and formation of more platelets, a number of factors are released that can be beneficial for the healing process of ailments when the PRP is reintroduced to the system. Some of these factors are platelet-derived growth factor isomers, vascular endothelial growth factor isomers, transforming growth factor isomers, and epithelial growth factor. Don't worry if you do not understand exactly what these terms mean! The only thing you really need to know is that these factors have been shown to have a number of beneficial impacts, including anti-inflammatory properties and immunomodulation aspects.

PRP And Cancer

PRP therapy for cancer is when the blood of a cancer patient has been taken, spun in a centrifuge, with the plasma then separated. The plasma is then injected into cancer patients in order to increase stem cell growth. Some practitioners state that this increases the macrophages, which are the specialised cells that come from white blood cells which contribute to the detection and destruction of harmful organisms and bacteria such as cancer cells. The belief is that the increase in macrophage will help to eat up the bad cells in the body – aiding in cancer cell death. Stem cells help the body's own cells to fight cancer by engineering a cancer-fighting immune system.

Some research has shown that PRP may also have some negative effects when one takes into consideration some of its effects on the immune system. As mentioned previously in the book, our body naturally produces immune cells known as T cells which actively fight cancer cells. Some studies have shown that PRP has been seen to directly suppress immune cells such as these, hindering them from performing their anti-cancer functions. Platelets have also been shown to protect cancer cells by giving them a sort of armour which consists of them transferring certain factors from the inside to the outside of the tumour cell, inhibiting the cytotoxic cell activity which would kill them.

Contrary to this, another piece of research has found that PRP administration has been able to kick-start the reversing of fibroblasts* in certain types of cancer such as breast cancer, which is an extremely important factor for the survival of the cell. Also when it comes to mouse-models, it was shown that a PRP gel was effective in decreasing cancer growth when compared to the control group. However, it was unclear as to how it was able to do this as the researchers were unable to find a difference in cellular morphology between the two groups, increasing the need for further research.

*An abstract from the nature.com website describes fibroblasts as the cockroaches of the human body. They survive severe stress that is usually lethal to all other cells, and they *are the only normal cell type that can be live-cultured from post-mortem and decaying tissue. Their resilient adaptation may reside in their intrinsic survival programmes and cellular plasticity.*

In a different animal study, PRP was administered alongside something known as BCG, or Bacillus Calmette-Guerin. The results were that about 70% of the animals injected showed a better histopathological recovery from certain types of lesions and increased certain immunoreceptors, thus aiding recovery.

PRP has also been shown to be a good way of stimulating tissue reconstruction as the contained cytokines and growth factors are able to stimulate stem cell production within a given tissue. This may make it a viable option to use in repair methods such as post-tumour removal surgeries, especially in those cases where a large chunk of tissue had to be removed and the healing of the surrounding areas may be impaired due to loss of blood flow. However, when it comes to research, this again has been shown to be an area of ambiguity.

Further research has shown that in certain instances, PRP could potentially have a negative effect by releasing certain growth factors that can potentially contribute to cancer growth over time. The process by which it does this is known as angiogenesis, which is when it both inhibits and stimulates. The exact mechanism by which it achieves this is still relatively unknown and so further research is required.

The Verdict

There is some promising research that shows there is a possibility that when PRP is combined with other treatments it may have beneficial outcomes and as described above, it can increase macrophage (Greek for 'big eaters') which are capable of eating damaged or diseased cells. As you have read, some of the research shows that, due to its ability to release growth factors, there is a possibility that it may accelerate some tumour growth and may be seen as counterproductive.

When it comes to making decisions in relation to incorporating PRP into your healing plan, it is definitely advised that you speak with your alternative or integrated cancer specialist and that you carry out your own research and make your decision based on what feels right for you.

My Mother's Journey

My mum had an alternative therapist that would come to our home and administer various treatments. One of these treatments was PRP. He would come 2 x per week and take my mum's blood, centrifuge it, and then reinject the plasma into her buttock. He believed that the PRP would increase the macrophage that would circulate in her system, as discussed earlier, which would then aid in eating up the cancer cells and toxins that are released .

****

Chapter Seven

Gerson Therapy And Colonic Hydrotherapy

Gerson Therapy

Gerson therapy is a type of diet regimen that consists of only eating a nutritious, organic, vegetarian diet while taking several supplements and enemas to boost health.

The therapy was first created by a doctor called Max Gerson who developed it in Germany between 1920 and 1930. Originally he did not design the regimen for cancer treatments but rather because he suffered from acute migraines that were inhibiting his standard of living. After following the diet for a while, Gerson claimed that he was able to completely cure his migraine issues and therefore postulated whether his treatment would be effective for other types of diseases. Eventually, he used it with patients who suffered from a variety of ailments including tuberculosis and cancer, though the success rate of these treatments is unknown.

The theoretic idea behind Gerson therapy is that cancer and other conditions are a symptom of larger underlying issues in an unhealthy body. Therefore, the practice is tied around correcting this underlying issue by giving the body all of the vital vitamins, nutrients and minerals that it needs in order to reset itself. This can sometimes be referred to as detoxing and aims to achieve a metabolic state of equilibrium.

Many advocates of the Gerson therapy champion the fact that no pesticides can be used to grow the food which are consumed and that food is prepared in special iron pots and pans. The diet has to be strictly followed without exception to offer optimal results.

As part of the therapy, you are encouraged to drink at least 20lbs of fruit and veg juice daily, usually 1 juice every hour over a 13 hour period. It's important to note that vegetables should be juiced, rather than blended into smoothies. The Gerson method advocates the intake of various supplements which can vary dependent on practitioners. Some of the most common ones are iodine, vitamin A, vitamin C, flaxseed oil, pepsin, potassium, and CoQ10.

There are a lot of vital points in favour of Gerson therapy despite mainstream health practitioners often denying its viability. The use of flaxseed oil, for example, has been shown to increase the bioavailability of vitamin A and aid in its absorption. Vitamin A is vital for our health, as it aids in the body's ability to defend itself via the immune system (which has been shown as one of the major contributors in the fight against cancer). Another positive is the ingestion of vitamin C in high dosages. Vitamin C, like vitamin A, aids the function of the immune system. However, it does so at a much greater rate and has the ability to aid both the innate and adaptive immune systems. It is also a very powerful antioxidant that can help to reduce the number of free radicals (electron stealing elements that roam around your body damaging cells). According to Cancer.gov free radicals have the ability to cause damage to DNA and could play a role in the development of cancer.

Coffee enemas play a big role in Gerson therapy. These enemas are derived from coffee and are supposed to help aid the liver in breaking down various toxins by increasing the size of the bile duct within the liver. It has been shown in studies that coffee-based enemas also have the ability to help with pain symptoms associated with cancers found within the GI tract.

As part of this therapy, coffee enemas are highly encouraged. You can take enemas multiple times a week in order to obtain their benefits. Aside from the dilation of the liver, coffee enemas have been linked to relieving constipation, removing parasites from the digestive system, releasing toxins from your system, and even treating autoimmune diseases. Even though they have been used for decades there has not been a great deal of scientific study into coffee enemas.

Doctors at the University of Minnesota showed that coffee administered rectally stimulates an enzyme system in the liver, called glutathione S-transferase, to 600%-700% above normal activity levels. This enzyme reacts with free radicals (which cause cell damage) in the bloodstream and neutralises them. These substances are dissolved in the bile and released through the bile flow from the liver and gallbladder to be excreted through the intestinal tract.

According to the Gerson Institute, a patient coping with a chronic degenerative disease or an acute illness can achieve a number of benefits from the lowering of blood serum toxin levels achieved by regular administration of coffee enemas. The benefits can include:

> » Increased cell energy production;
> » Enhanced tissue health;
> » Improved blood circulation;
> » Better immunity and tissue repair; and
> » Cellular regeneration.

Another major part of Gerson therapy is the high consumption of potassium supplements as well as lower sodium intake. It is known that sodium and potassium have a major role to play when it comes to the body's ability to store and secrete water within the cells. During various experiments, Gerson found that diseased cells often had an excess of sodium and were low in potassium, while healthy cells had the opposite concentrations. According to research, electrolyte imbalances are highly common within cancer patients.

Gerson therapy appears to have many benefits and it seems to be foundationally correct in addressing many vitamin and mineral deficiencies. As is always the case, some people have reported adverse reactions to the Gerson diet, so be sure to investigate further to see if this is the right treatment for you or your loved one.

The cost associated with Gerson therapy can be quite expensive, however with the right amount of research you could potentially cut the overhead costs significantly. If you already have iron cookware and are close to a farmers market or have the ability to grow or purchase organic produce, then it should not be too difficult for you to treat yourself using the Gerson method should you choose to do so. I would advise having an initial consultation with a therapist to get you started.

As the main function of the Gerson therapy is to boost immunity, many of its practitioners do not advise that their patients engage in chemotherapy, as it is majorly disruptive to the immune system. They instead say that radiotherapy is a better alternative to use in conjunction with Gerson therapy.

So what do we make of all this and should you engage in the Gerson therapy? As you know, alternative treatments are not a 'one size fits all' scenario and it will depend on your situation. It may be that you have a chronic amount of sodium in your system as well as several nutritional deficiencies. Your cancer could also have been caused by pesticides which have been linked to cancer numerous times. If this is the case, then Gerson therapy may be a viable option for yours or your loved one's cancer treatment plan.

If you are pregnant or if you have any bleeding from your bowel, enemas are not recommended. It may also not be the best option if you already have problems in other areas, such as in the GI tract (IBS, constipation) or heart and lung problems. If you want to give the therapy a try, you should speak to a practitioner as well as your overseeing oncologist and integrative therapist in order to best determine your route of action.

Ms Shemila Tharani and Ms Penny Deadman of the Body Vibrant Clinic, Slough, UK, offer coffee enema treatments for clients that may initially feel uncomfortable administering them themselves. The Body Vibrant Clinic also offers various other therapies, including colon hydrotherapy, ozone enemas, rectal insufflation, hyperbaric oxygen therapy, far infrared and ozone saunas.

The Gerson institute website provides a list of the licenced Gerson centres where the treatment can take place: http://gerson.org/gerpress/.

Colonic Hydrotherapy

Colonic hydrotherapy or irrigation as it is sometimes known, in a nutshell is the cleaning out of waste material within the bowels using water. You will have a very small tube inserted into your rectum that allows for the flow of warm water which cleanses the inside of your colon. The therapy involves gentle, continual bathing of the colon by flushing warm filtered water into the rectum. This process enables the water to cleanse the large intestine, resulting in a gentle release.

The water flow triggers a response in which the patient begins to expel the water and waste through a tube that allows the therapist to monitor the expelled bowel contents. This response is known as peristalsis, which is a normal pattern of smooth muscle contractions that propel foodstuffs through the digestive tract. During the treatment, the therapist gently massages the patient's abdomen to help dislodge impacted matter.

Colonic hydrotherapy is recommended for some cancer patients as it can assist the body to expel any toxins that may have been caused by toxic overload. The treatment can help to speed up the process of which it expels any unwanted toxins. Colonic hydrotherapy also has a variety of other health benefits.

My Mother's Journey

In order to aid the detoxification process on the body and to help my mum to eliminate toxins, my mum has regular colonic hydrotherapy sessions.

****

Chapter Eight

Intravenous High Dose Vitamin C And Vitamin D

Vitamins can be introduced into the body in various ways and a common question is, why should a patient opt for the intravenous method of vitamins and minerals as opposed to oral form? The reason that IV vitamins and minerals are the preferred method is due to the fact that by introducing the vitamins directly into the vein, the vitamin compounds enter the blood stream immediately and can make its way to the cells that require it very quickly. If you choose to take these supplements orally, although still beneficial, the capsule needs to be processed via the digestive system which means that a lot of potency in the compound can be lost while going through this process. Also when a person is ill, their digestive system can become impaired, meaning that the IV route may be the best and most beneficial method for vitamin therapy.

High Dose Vitamin C – Oral Form

Vitamin C has been shown to impair cancer cell growth directly when given at very high doses. Vitamin C is one of the most popular vitamins that is known for supporting your immune system. If your immune system is working well, theoretically your body should have a better chance of working optimally and fighting off cancer cells.

Many of us are familiar with vitamin C being ingested orally, however, it has been shown numerously that absorption into the body through this method is quite low and that up to 95% of the vitamin C is excreted through your urine. There is another way to take vitamin C and this is in the form of liposomal vitamin C, which is especially formulated for high doses. Liposomes are a type of phospholipid, which have very small carrier spheres. These carrier spheres allow the vitamin C to be transported directly through intracellular pathways directly into the bloodstream.

If intravenous vitamin C is not an option, the next best thing would be to get your high dosage through liposomal vitamin C.

High Dose Vitamin C - Intravenous Therapy

Many studies have shown that the best way for high doses of vitamin C to be given is via the intravenous method, which delivers the compound directly into the bloodstream.

Dr Chen, from the National Institute of Diabetes and Digestive and Kidney Diseases, carried out a clinical in vitro study that showed a direct link between vitamin C injections and cancer cell death. Research was conducted on a variety of cancer cells, some of which were human and others being animal cells. It was found within the study that vitamin C was able to kill the cancer cells at a dosage far lower than what was required to kill normal cells.

An abstract taken from Sciencedaily.com states that clinical trials found it is safe to regularly infuse brain and lung cancer patients with 800-1,000 times the daily recommended amount of vitamin C as a possible strategy to improve outcomes of standard cancer treatments. In work presented in Cancer Cell in March 2017, University of Iowa researchers showed pathways by which altered iron metabolism in cancer cells and not normal cells led to increased sensitivity to cancer cell death caused by high dose vitamin C.

Some doctors prefer to treat their patients with up to 100,000mg of vitamin C intravenously instead of chemotherapy which in comparison to the RDA of 120mg, is a huge jump. Many alternative health doctors are astounded at the RDA for vitamin C as there are incredible benefits to be had if you intake a higher dosage.

A study by a group of scientists in USC and the IFOM Cancer Institute in Milan found that a combination of fasting and high dose vitamin C was effective at treating some aggressive colorectal cancer in mice. The researchers were aware that fasting could be challenging for some patients, so suggested a more feasible option of a low calorie plant-based diet, which causes the body to believe that it's in a fasting state. Once this state is reached, it is recommended that high dose vitamin C is infused.

Many cancer patients are aware of this treatment and have started to include high dose vitamin C therapy into their treatment plan as it yields great results for a lot of cancer sufferers. I would definitely recommend speaking to your alternative or integrated cancer specialist to see if this can be incorporated into your routine.

Vitamin D

Vitamin D should not be forgotten, as a deficiency of vitamin D is linked to an increase in adults developing cancer. Breast cancer survival is also linked to vitamin D status. Researchers have also shown that optimal levels of vitamin D may prevent various kinds of cancer from forming and or metastasising.

Vitamin D is free; 10-15 minutes of unprotected sun exposure between 11:00-13:00 is recommended for colon cancer and heart disease patients.

Harvard University carried out randomised trials, testing the results of vitamin D on postmenopausal women. The women took 1,100 international units (IU) of vitamin D daily alongside 1,400 to 1,500 milligrams of calcium per day. The findings were that the supplementation of vitamin D and calcium reduced their risk of developing non-skin related cancers after 4 years by 77%.

Once again, use your own judgment and research in relation to how much sun exposure is safe for you in your healing journey.

My Mother's Journey

My mum was not too keen on taking vitamin C as she said it made her feel as though she was overheating. She therefore took as much vitamin C orally that she could manage and then started to take liposomal vitamin C when we realised it was the better option.

▶

Try to take it in the purest form possible, as many supplements are full of nasty unnecessary additives that bulk it up, such as propylene glycol, cellulose, titanium dioxide, stearic acid, magnesium stearate, silicon dioxide, starch, and the list goes on.

My mum also takes a vitamin D supplement daily and makes sure that she spends a minimum of 15 minutes in direct sunlight each day.

****

Chapter Nine

Ozone Therapy For Cancer:
What It Does To The Body

We are about to enter a different kind of world when it comes to alternative cancer treatments. This next treatment shows huge promise when it comes to helping people in their fight against cancer.

This therapy is relatively undiscovered in the western world and I think that it is time for people to see the full capacity of this treatment and how it can positively influence their healing journey.

A Brief History

Ozone was first discovered in the middle of the 19th century and is unique in its molecular structure. Ozone, which is O3, differs from its cousin, oxygen, which is O2. This is because it has three oxygen atoms rather than just two. Ozone has been used for a variety of different reasons over the decades but has been in use pretty much since its discovery. Early practitioners used ozone to disinfect drinking water by using its antibacterial properties. It is a little known secret that famous scientist and inventor, Nikola Tesla, was actually the first to patent an ozone-generating machine before the turn of the last century. He even created a company known as the Tesla Ozone Company, however, his project never really took off.

During WWI, physicians treating wounded soldiers were using ozone as a topical agent in order to disinfect wounds and for anti-inflammatory purposes. Later in the 1980s, there was a rumour going around that it may be useful for treating HIV as a couple of German scientists had found that ozone was effective in vitro (which means testing has been performed on a non-living organism). It was, however, later discovered that in vivo (which means testing has been performed on a living organism i.e. on an animal or human) the treatment was not effective.

Between 1980 and 1995 ozone was widespread and used for a long list of different things, including acne, allergies, cerebral sclerosis, gangrene, burns, gastric cancer, eczema, open sores, and wound healing in general.

Current Usage

Ozone is usually kept in its gaseous form and has no smell or colour to speak of.

Within nature ozone is usually found in our atmosphere where it shields living organisms on Earth from harmful UV radiation. It has to be mentioned that many people believe ozone to be dangerous and without medical use. Certain studies have even shown that ozone can be extremely harmful to the lungs and respiratory system when it is found within smog. The FDA banned its use within the United States in 2003 and claimed that:

"Ozone is a toxic gas with no known useful medical application in specific, adjunctive, or preventive therapy."

Many scientific studies, data and researchers would deny this claim and are in full support of ozone as a potential treatment for a variety of different ailments, including cancer. Up until recently, it has been difficult to fully study the effects of ozone as the technology needed to generate medical concentrates of the substance was lacking. However, now that they are available, research is being conducted globally on an ongoing basis.

Ozone is currently used in medicine throughout the world for a variety of different ailments, including bacterial infections, viral infections, and immunosuppressant diseases. In most cases, the gas is administered in a very safe dosage and a therapeutic manner in accordance with proven and safe methodologies. For example, it is never given via inhalation (for the reasons outlined above) and the preferred method of administration is rectal or intravenously.

Many European countries use ozone therapy freely. In Germany, over 7,000 doctors use it daily. Ozone is placed in ambulances to help to treat stroke victims, as the incidence of permanent paralysis is reduced when ozone therapy is administered. Russia is another country that endorses the use of ozone for medicinal purposes.

But how exactly does ozone work? We already covered what it is good for but when undergoing treatment, it is always good to know the mechanism by which a specific treatment is working. Ozone essentially helps to deactivate bacteria and viruses. It does this by compromising the security of the cells within the bacteria or virus by oxidising the lipids on proteins. In viruses specifically, ozone disrupts its reproductive cycle, inhibiting proliferation.

Ozone also has the ability to stimulate and increase the glycolysis rate within red blood cells. This, in short, leads to greater oxygen metabolism within cells and tissues within the body. It also has the ability to stimulate ATP production, which is basically an energy molecule that your cells burn in order to do the work that they need to do. Think of ATP as fuel for your cells. In this way, ozone has the ability to increase the energy output of cells, making them better at doing their usual job.

In order to fight infection and viruses, it is also important to have a great amount of blood flow to a given area, which carries all the nutrients and cofactors needed for repair. Ozone also aids in this specific process as it produces something known as prostacyclin, which is a known vasodilator. A vasodilator increases the size of your blood vessels by helping them to relax, therefore allowing more regular blood flow through them.

In relation to cancer, you may have heard that cancer cells do not like oxygen (once again this may be referred to as quackery), so by using ozone therapy you are effectively flooding the body with oxygen and theoretically encouraging apoptosis, which is cancer cell death.

Ozone In Cancer Treatment

Ozone may play a critical role in a number of different ways when it comes to its ability to aid against cancer and tumours. The first and often most widely known is the fact that it benefits the immune system. As mentioned earlier in the book, the immune system produces T cells, which are critical in fighting cancer. When ozone is given at a dosage of around 55 μg/cc, it generates the production of something known as interferon. These are a group of proteins whose purpose it is to signal during infections. It is basically the body's way of warning itself when it is under threat. So if a cell is infected with something it will release interferons, which will then signal to other cells that they need to upregulate their own defences as to not become infected. Interferons also activate a certain type of immune cell: the T cells.

When it comes to cancer treatment specifically, there may be an even more impressive feat for ozone and that is the fact that, at the dosage listed above, it has the ability to pump out a large amount of tumour necrosis factor. As the name so explains, tumour necrosis factor is a signalling protein that has the ability to cause apoptosis. In layman's terms, this means that it has the ability to kill cells. Various studies have found that a dysregulation of this important protein has been inexplicably linked with cancer (as well as some other degenerative diseases, such as Alzheimer's).

These are just the indirect benefits of ozone. When it comes to a possible therapy for cancer, several studies have shown that ozone can directly damage the cell walls of tumours as well as elevate the effects of other treatments, such as chemotherapy. Examples of these studies span back over the decades. One of the earlier ones was conducted in 1980 and was published in the well-known journal *Science*. In this study it was shown that ozone had the ability to inhibit the growth of cancer cells within human tissue without it impacting non-cancerous cells. The tissues examined were lung, breast, and uterus tissues. Another study released a decade later in 1990 showed that ozone had an empowering effect on 5FU (5-fluorouracil) within breast and colon tumours. 5FU is one of the most widely used and prescribed drugs taken by cancer patients. The results were somewhat replicated in 2017 by another study which showed that it not only had the ability to boost the effect of 5FU but also of cisplatin, which is a common chemotherapy drug.

It should be noted, however, that these studies were conducted in a laboratory setting rather than in clinics and were delivered in vitro. When clinics that provide ozone treatment give you ozone, the delivery mechanism for the tumour is quite different to what has been shown in these studies.

Ozone therapy is certainly more than promising and can be used in conjunction with various other treatments with no ill effects. Ozone therapy may be a great option for you and is definitely worth looking into to see if you can use it to enhance your treatment.

How To Get Therapy:

Now that you know more about ozone, you may be wondering how you can actually receive ozone therapy and what options for treatment there are available. For the sake of this book, we will focus on three specific methods which people can utilise in order to receive ozone therapy.

Autohemotherapy And The 10 Pass Method

Autohemotherapy is a type of treatment in which the patient's blood is drawn, infused with ozone, and then this is reinfused back into the patient. The way this is usually done is by placing the patient's blood within a special concealment bag with an anti-regulatory drug, such as heparin, and then mixing the blood with medicinal ozone. Initially, 200ml of blood is drawn from a patient, which is then infused with 70 mcg/ml of ozone and then reinfused back into the patient while being under a max pressure of 0.8bar.

There are two ways to perform this therapy. One is by normobaric MAH, which uses the force of gravity to both withdraw and re-inject blood. After the patient is given a blood thinning injection, the blood is drawn into the bag when it is lower than the patient's arm and then re-infused back into the patient with the bag above the patient's arm. Gravity is used to aid either the blood flow into the bag, or from the bag back into the patient's arm.

The second way to perform this therapy is hyperbaric MAH, which is when the blood is drawn from the patient into a bottle using a vacuum and once in the bottle, it is mixed with an anti-coagulant, either sodium citrate or heparin, to prevent the blood from clotting. The machine creates both negative (vacuum) and positive (hyperbaric) pressure, which will assist with the blood flow back into the body.

Dr Lahodny is a well-renowned pioneer of multiple, or 10 pass, ozone therapy, which is the same as the regular treatment but instead relies on creating super high concentrations of ozone within a person's blood. Dr Lahodny's method involves repeating the above method 10 times, where a total of 2,000ml of blood is drawn and combined with 2,000ml of ozone. This gives a combined and total dosage of 140,000mcg. Dr Lahodny believes that this dose of ozone stimulates your body's release of stem cells. He has also reported in his own research that the high dose upticks the production of ATP energy in red cells by 500 %.

Dr Robert Rowen is another doctor who uses the 10 pass ozone method on cancer patients. He trained with Dr Lahodny to learn the 10 pass method and utilises the treatment with patients who have chronic illnesses and diseases, yielding great results from this therapy. He has his own clinic, along with Dr Terri Su, in Santa Barbara and offers innovative biologic treatments.

Dr Akbar Khan, Director of The Medicor Cancer Centre in Canada, personally trains his staff on how to administer this method. The medicor.com website says that ozone has been extensively researched, with hundreds of peer-reviewed scientific publications available that demonstrate the effectiveness of ozone in treating many different diseases, including cancer, autoimmune disease, inflammatory conditions, cardiovascular disease, endocrine disease, chronic pain, and acute or chronic infections. There is even evidence that ozone can help to slow the aging process. The best part is that ozone has almost no side effects when used correctly. Medicor's own staff members have experienced the healing ability of ozone first-hand.

The biggest known side effect of receiving ozone treatment in this manner is that it relies on very large doses of heparin to stop the blood from coagulating. Such dosages as those administered during the 10 pass method have been shown to potentially cause several side effects, so this should be investigated further should you be interested in this method.

There are currently two such hyperbaric ozone machines on the market: the Zotzmann Ozon 2000 and the Herrmann Hyper Medozon Comfort. When embarking on my research for cancer therapies, I contacted Dr Zotzmann personally who provided me with help, contacts, and support in relation to ozone therapy. His kindness really spurred me on to continue my research into this field. This reminded me that human kindness does still exist and if you reach out to people, you may be surprised at the help and support that is offered to you.

If you decide to go ahead with an ozone treatment it could potentially be expensive. However, the alternative to autohemotherapy ozone is intestinal/rectal ozone therapy, which has a reasonable price tag per treatment. Alternatively, with proper research and practice, you can learn to administer this treatment yourself at home.

Intestinal/Rectal Ozone Therapy

Rectal ozone therapy is when ozone is inserted through the rectum. A machine is used to create the ozone and then passed through via a catheter into the rectum for the gas to be absorbed through the intestinal walls into the bloodstream. For intestinal/rectal insufflations, the colon should be cleared out by means of a colonic or an enema with ozonated water to prevent eliminated toxins from being reabsorbed.

When delivering rectal ozone, the gas needs to be delivered very slowly in order to circumvent any negative effects on the colon. In the presence of oxygen, bad bacteria, candida, and yeast in the large intestine may form gas and cause temporary bloating. It is therefore advised that, when taking rectal insufflation, probiotics should be taken in order to support the gut flora.

Multiple pass ozone therapy can be delivered rectally however, the process will take a much longer period of time and may be fairly uncomfortable for the patient. This option is available and the most economical.

Hyperbaric Oxygen

We briefly mentioned the use of hyperbaric oxygen in relation to ozone treatment. This technique is when you are administered 100% oxygen to breathe while under high atmospheric pressures which has actually been proven to have a host of health benefits in its own right.

This treatment is done in an enclosed space such as a capsule or a pressure room and you will be asked by your practitioner to breathe pure oxygen through ventilating tubes which you place around your neck and on your nostrils. It can also be done with a mask. The premise behind this treatment is that, under pressure, the absorption of gases into human tissues is increased greatly. Often, our body finds it difficult to transport oxygen, which is desperately needed in wound healing and also eliminating cancer, to the infected area. In this regard, the hyperbaric oxygen treatment bypasses the need for oxygen transport in the conventional sense by pumping the body full of oxygen. As cancer cells use glucose to survive, saturating them with oxygen may also have some benefits against tumours in this manner.

More and more people are realising the potential benefits of this alternative treatment and it may be one of the most effective yet when it comes to cancer treatment. While you do not have to get mega dosages of ozone, it may certainly be worth your time to research further or speak to a clinic that provides ozone treatments.

MEDLINE (the largest medical database in the world) contains information on published ozone research. This database can be searched by anyone interested in finding medical ozone therapy publications. A collection of over 2,000 ozone research papers from around the world are available on this web-based database: Zotero ISCO3 Ozone.

My Mother's Journey

Upon initial diagnosis, our local MS charity allowed my mum access to use their oxygen chambers on a regular basis.

After investigating ozone via the blood (autohemotherapy), which is most effective, we realised that it was not an option for my mum as her veins would not allow this to be carried out. However, I found out that you can still get ozone into the body rectally. Some people deem it not as effective, but it is a treatment that I feel is quite efficient at delivering the extra molecule of oxygen to the body.

Rectal ozone is a longer, more drawn out process, but it does mean that ozone is being received into the body. I bought the equipment required and was taught how to carry this out . I then trained my stepdad on how to work the machine so that they could administer this every other day when possible. A probiotic is required when carrying out regular rectal ozone in order to keep the gut balance correct. There are several YouTube videos that show you how to do this method but remember you should always seek professional training in the first instance.

▶

Ozone therapy was delivered, at first, 2 x a week and up to every other day. 1 pass ozone rectally is the equivalent of a litre/1,000 ml. Some doctors recommend 10 pass ozone for cancer patients or those with advanced disease, however my mum cannot take the dose required and can get up to 750ml per treatment max as she has a sensitive bowel. The perk of doing this at home is that she can do it as often as she is able to and in an inexpensive way.

****

Chapter Ten

DCA, Hydrogen Peroxide, And DMSO For Cancer

Cancer can be attacked and approached from a number of different angles, as we have already discussed in this book. You may want to encourage the immune system to fight your cancer or use different treatments that attack the cancer more directly. One methodology we have not yet approached in detail is the eradication of cancer from its metabolic approach. Every cancer cell, just as regular cells, have a metabolism which they need to stay alive and therefore it is possible to target that mechanism in order to promote the death of cancer cells.

This is where DCA, or dichloroacetate, comes in. In the past, this medication has been used in various different scenarios, including lactic acidosis, errors within mitochondrial metabolism and diabetes. In the last ten years or so, it has also become quite well known as an anti-cancer drug. It is an analogue of acetic acid and is usually administered in dosage ranges of about 50-200mg. These dosages have been shown to effectively decrease the size of cancerous growths as well as their ability to proliferate. It has actually been shown in studies carried out by Tataranni and Piccoli (2019) that DCA has the direct ability to eliminate cancer cells as well as their mitochondrial respiratory capacity.

DCA works on the metabolism of the cancer cell. Cancer cells are known to have an increase in glycolysis, which converts glucose into energy, when compared to normal cells. This leads to an overproduction of something known as lactate, which can then be taken in by the surrounding cells, enhancing tumour cancer growth.

DCA forces cancer cells to shift their metabolic preference from glycolysis to oxidation (using oxygen for energy) by blocking something known as PDK, which in turn, then blocks another molecule known as PDH. While it may be difficult to remember all the acronyms, it is not that important. The simple explanation is the fact that when PDH is activated, it is able to disrupt the metabolic advantage that tumour cells have. This escalates into a number of different factors within the cell that consequently results in the death of the cancer cell.

While all of this may sound amazing to anyone who is struggling with cancer, there are several factors to keep in mind before asking your doctor if you can engage in this treatment. There are several GI-related side effects that have been reported with the ingestion of DCA, which means that if you also suffer from bowel problems it may not be the best option for you. It has also been found that DCA can potentially cause peripheral neuropathy. This is the damage and consequent pain associated with damaged nerves in the peripheral nervous system (everything apart from your brain and spinal cord). It has been theorised that this is because the DCA causes overloading of the mitochondria, your cell's energy centres, which then, in turn, blocks your body's ability to properly produce antioxidants, which are vital for a number of different functions. Therefore, many practitioners advise that extrinsic sources of antioxidants are administered with DCA treatment.

We have mentioned in the conventional treatment chapter of this book the fact that cancer drugs are often used in synergy in order to prevent the cancer cells from adapting to any one drug and therefore avoiding apoptosis. DCA is a great drug to use in combination with other chemotherapeutic agents in this manner. It has been shown that this combination enhances the efficiency of which chemotherapy drugs operate and also minimises toxicity risks. If you are currently receiving traditional chemotherapy, it may be wise for you to speak to your overseeing clinician about the possibility of adding DCA into your regimen. The FDA have not approved the use of DCA for cancer treatment, so please ensure that you talk to your alternative healthcare practitioner should you be interested in this treatment.

Dr Akbar Khan, Director of the Medicor Cancer Clinic, is one of the leading authorities in the field and has provided a lot of research in regards to DCA. For further reference to his work, please visit www.medicorcancercentre.com and see the reference list for more details.

Hydrogen Peroxide

When compared to DCA, hydrogen peroxide is definitely seen more as an alternative route for treating cancer. HP is a compound that finds its uses in many different areas of life, including disinfecting cuts and whitening teeth. The premise of the compound as a treatment for cancer comes from the assumption that low levels of blood oxygen can be the causality for many cancers and therefore HP, which is known as an oxygenating compound, can kill cancer cells by overloading them with oxygen.

As mentioned previously, cancer cells use glucose to produce their energy while normal cells use oxygen. This has become known as the Warburg effect. And so, based on this premise, the idea of using oxygen to eliminate cancer was born. This theory has experienced backing from the scientific community since its inception. All the way back in the 1950s, a rodent study found that 60% of rats who had cancerous growths were completely cancer-free after 60 days of drinking hydrogen peroxide. However, subsequent studies that attempted to directly inject the tumours with the compound found that it was not effective at destroying cancer, and some more modern research seems to have thrown a wrench into the realm of hydrogen peroxide, as it was found in some studies that cancer cells can survive with or without oxygen.

I have come across several stories where cancer patients have used HP therapy as part of their protocol by diluting 4 cups of 35% concentrated hydrogen peroxide into a bath. Once again, I would advise that you speak with yours or your loved one's integrative oncologist before starting any therapy involving hydrogen peroxide, as there have been several stories of improper use and severe side effects have been known to accompany this treatment.

The research is fairly inconclusive at this moment in time so it's up to you to make the right decisions based on the research that you conduct.

DMSO For Cancer

DMSO is a natural liquid derived from trees. It is a by-product of paper manufacturing. DMSO is also a solvent that is used to mix certain drugs into water, even though they may be insoluble in water. It is also used as a carrier to bring drugs into the body through the skin. DMSO is currently approved as a preservative for bone marrow and organ transplants and for treatment of a bladder disease called interstitial cystitis. It is also a generic drug (not patentable), which means there is little interest among drug manufacturers in researching it as a treatment for cancer and other diseases, because of its low profit potential.

There are many publications on DMSO dating back to the 1960s. DMSO has been found to be effective as a cancer treatment, a pain treatment, a treatment for inflammation and a treatment for brain swelling due to head injury. DMSO reduces swelling by removing water from cells and reducing water leakage from blood vessels in tumours. It does not have a 'rebound effect' when it is stopped (no sudden worsening of symptoms), unlike steroid medication such as dexamethasone, which has side effects such as muscle loss, immune suppression and stomach ulceration.

DMSO appears to reduce the risk of seizures, as long as no overdose is given and works as a cancer therapy by promoting differentiation (a process of transforming primitive rapidly growing cells into more normal-behaving cells that do not grow). DMSO also has been demonstrated to stimulate a tumour suppressor protein called HLJ1, which reduces tumour cell invasion and metastases.

Several publications demonstrate that DMSO works in a variety of cancers. In lab studies DMSO has been shown to work as a cancer treatment for melanoma, colon cancer, leukaemia, lung cancer, ovarian cancer and lymphoma.

There are 2 published human intravenous DMSO cancer studies by Dr Hoang and his colleagues: one for prostate cancer and one for gallbladder/bile duct cancer. In these studies, DMSO was combined with sodium bicarbonate (baking soda) and administered by intravenous infusion up to 5 days per week. These studies demonstrated significant improvement in clinical symptoms, blood tests, and quality of life. There were no major side effects from the infusions.

In the bile duct cancer study of 9 patients, there was relief of bile duct obstruction, improvement of liver function and the 6 month progression-free survival was 100% (the cancer stabilised for 6 months in all patients). The duration of the study was only 6 months, so it is possible that the benefits of therapy would continue for a longer period.

In the prostate cancer study of 18 patients, 8 were newly diagnosed and 10 had been treated previously but conventional therapy had failed. All patients had metastases to the bones. After 1.5 months of therapy, all patients experienced over 30% reduction of their pain scores and none of the 6 patients who needed morphine before therapy needed to continue it. There was improvement of fatigue in 78% of patients, improvement in urine flow in 83%, improvement in spinal cord compression in 60%, and improvement in urinary bleeding and swelling in 100% (of those that experienced these issues before therapy). The only side effects noted were mild headache or chills during the infusion, which could be prevented by slowing down the infusion.

It is important to note that the benefits of therapy persisted after DMSO infusions were stopped. This indicates that the therapy was not simply controlling symptoms (like pain medication) but had effectively treated the cancer. Based on the existing published research and our own experience, it appears DMSO may work on any cancer type.

The website http://www.dmso.org/ is full of information on DMSO. It was created by Dr Stanley Jacob, one of the world experts on DMSO, and a physician who was heavily involved in DMSO research from the 1960s.

MEDLINE (the largest medical database in the world) contains information on published DMSO cancer research. This database can be searched by anyone interested in finding DMSO publications.

Details on DMSO have been shared by the Medicor Cancer Centre website.

My Mum's Story

My mum's alternative therapist used to administer DMSO intravenously on a weekly basis. Unfortunately, the doctor was unable to perform home visits after some time, and my mum was encouraged to take DMSO in oral form instead. She did not like taking this orally, so she ceased including DMSO in her protocol. We are however, looking at ways to reintroduce this back into her healing plan.

****

Chapter Eleven

Herbal Medicine And Hoxsey Treatment

For a very long time now, herbal medicine has been practiced not only as an alternative type of medicine but also in complementary and comprehensive treatments for all kinds of ailments. As cancer is one of the most common and difficult diseases, it is safe to assume many people have looked into herbs and their benefits for cancer patients, and many of them doing it are caregivers to said patients. When it comes to herbal medicine, there are various herbs that can be used in teas and tinctures to help strengthen our bodies and enhance their ability to fight disease.

While it can be relatively easy to find herbs that are supposed to improve the way your body works or ease cancer symptoms, most doctors advise their cancer patients to stay away from herbs as they can interfere with chemotherapy treatments. I think that the reasoning behind this is because herbs and natural sources of medicine are not taught to doctors studying at medical school. They focus only on what is FDA regulated and sold by big pharmaceutical companies and unfortunately, a lot of the herbs and natural sources of treatment are not beneficial to the governments from a financial perspective.

Due to the lack of education on natural supplementation, I think that there is a huge gap in the treatment plans of patients and the reason as to why pharmaceutical drugs are widely used and natural medicines and herbs are shunned.

Many doctors have not been exposed to the knowledge and are genuinely unaware of how these wonderful sources of nature have the ability to cure. Because of this, there are not many studies on what the exact components of specific herbs are available to them as per their curriculum and there is not enough data, if any, shown to them, for them to see how these herbs would impact the body when taken alongside chemotherapeutic agents. Because of this, many western physicians are not of much help when it comes to giving advice on alternative natural treatments, as they do not have placebo studies or evidence available to them that show the effects that take place when chemo drugs are used alongside various herbs and supplements. Because of this, they will advise you to not use them.

You can, however, find integrative oncologists that can provide you with a wealth of knowledge on natural supplementations that you can take as part of your protocol and who can advise you on the various herbs that can support cancer patients.

Hoxsey Formula

When first embarking on my cancer research journey, I found information on a herbal tincture called the Hoxsey formula, that claimed to have properties with the ability to shrink tumours.

Harry Hoxsey's great grandfather developed the Hoxsey herbal tonic when his horse seemed to have been cured of his leg tumour after eating some wild herbs. The herbs were later combined with some popular cancer remedies.

Throughout the first half of the 20th century, Hoxsey's remedies were being promoted through his clinic and newspaper but, eventually, he was stopped from selling them by the US government because he didn't have a medical license.

Hoxsey claims that the tonic stimulates the detoxification of the body and normalises cell metabolism. While there is no scientific proof for his claim as there were no trials used to prove it, the American Cancer Society advises cancer patients not to use it. Hoxsey also claimed that his topical remedy can target skin cancer cells and kill them, but the ingredients known in the remedy are also known to burn healthy tissue.

The Hoxsey herbal therapy is available at clinics in Tijuana, Mexico, however, it is currently illegal in the US due to the lack of evidence supporting the treatment for cancer use and the side effects associated with it. The therapy consists of restrictive diets and herbal tonics.

Harry Hoxsey's 'brown' tonic contains liquorice, red clover, potassium iodide, burdock root, barberry, stillingia root, pokeweed, cascara, prickly ash bark, and buckthorn bark. The diet part involves eliminating a series of items: vinegar, tomatoes, pork, carbonated drinks, alcohol, sugar, salt and bleached flour. The Hoxsey protocol encourages the supplementation of calcium, iron, vitamin C, grape juice and yeast. With this therapy, Hoxsey claims that the treatment will detoxify the body, balance body chemistry and strengthen the immune system.

Hoxsey claimed that the internal formulation 'stimulates the elimination of toxins that poison the system, thereby correcting the abnormal blood chemistry and normalising cell metabolism.' His head nurse also added that it normalises metabolism, restores acid/base balance and restores the normal immune function. Studies have been conducted on the individual components of the tonic such as red clover, liquorice, burdock, pokeroot, stillingia and barberry, and the results indicated possible anti-tumour and immune system stimulation properties, but the concentration in the tonic and the way that they work together has not been determined.

There are several side effects listed from the ingredients, however despite this, the Bio-Medical Center in Tijuana, Mexico, claims their success rate to be between 50-85% in their promotional material and the Director of the Bio-Medical Center, Mildred Nelson, has publicly claimed a success rate of 80%.

Because of its claims and the anecdotal evidence of its success, there is a need for more peer-reviewed medical and scientific research for the treatment and its potential effectiveness against cancer. I also think that this treatment may not be as effective now as it may have been when Hoxsey first made the formula as we are exposed to far more chemicals, pesticides, and processed products than ever before. However some people have got some great results from this tonic.

You can find different medical herbalists worldwide who are fully trained in the science of herbal medicine. Each herbalist will have their own approach as to what herbs should be included in your holistic cancer treatment plan.

Dr Robert Morse is the creator and founder of God's Herbs, Dr Morse's Herbal Health Club, and the International School of Detoxification. He has degrees in Naturopathy, Naturopathic Medicine, Biochemistry, Iridology, Herbology, Nutrition, and Fitness. He is a popular Master Herbalist and more details on how herbs can assist with your healing can be found at https://www.drmorsesherbalhealthclub. Dr Morse's Herbal Health Club is free to join and gives you access to a large amount of free information, as well as the ability to order very high quality herbal formulas. He also has a lot of videos on YouTube that are informative and easy to understand.

I think that it's wise to talk to an alternative cancer therapist and herbalist before purchasing any herbs yourself as it's important to buy herbs that do not counteract or affect any treatment plan or medication that you, or your loved one, may be on.

There are several natural substances that are tested in the RGCC test (discussed later in the book), the test results will show you how effective various herbs work at killing your particular cancer. Some of the natural substances tested that can be discussed with your herbalist dependent on your results are:

» Mistletoe;

» Boswellia Serratta;

» Algaricus Blazei Murill;

» Artecin.

Your herbalist will know how to add any recommended herbs into your protocol.

My Mother's Journey

Upon initial diagnosis, my mum saw an integrated cancer specialist who prescribed her a tincture that he deemed was better than the Hoxsey tincture, however, she was unable to stomach the mixture. She also initially used a variety of Dr Morse's Herbs to help her to detoxify and support her organs.

Later in her journey, when my mum was diagnosed with cachexia, we enlisted the help of another herbalist who prescribed her various supplements and powders to help her to gain weight, restore and rebalance her hormones, and boost her immune system.

****

Chapter Twelve

Hyper/Hypothermia,

Infrared Saunas, And Light Therapy

Hyper/Hypothermia

Hyperthermia, in terms of cancer treatment, refers to a state in which high heat is used to attack cancer cells. Hypothermia is the opposite, when extremely low temperatures are used, and can also be referred to as cryosurgery.

Hyper/Hypothermia is not usually used as a standalone treatment for cancer but instead as a conjunctive treatment with something such as radiation therapy. The temperatures used for this treatment vary, but usually do not exceed -50 degrees for hypothermia and 45 degrees Celsius (113F) for hyperthermia. Certain research studies have shown that intense temperatures have the ability to cause cell death within cancer by damaging their proteins and destroying other structures within the cells. This makes it a good option to use in conjunction with conventional treatments, as it has been shown in numerous studies to increase their effectiveness significantly.

Hyperthermia treatment can be given in a variety of ways and depends on where your tumour is located. Cancer growths on or near the surface of the skin can have high heat applied directly to them, while tumours hidden deep within the body may require something known as an interstitial treatment. In the latter, a number of needles are inserted into the tumour while the patient is under general anaesthetic. Then, using radio waves, the needles are heated to high temperatures, allowing the cancer cells to be killed. For external treatment, patients usually do not have to be under general anaesthetic.

Cryosurgery works in a very similar way when it comes to external cancer applications. Usually, liquid nitrogen is used to cool the affected area and freeze the tumour, thereby killing the cancer cells. For internal tumours, hollow probes are inserted into the tumour and the liquid nitrogen is then circulated through the probe, cooling it and the surrounding area (the cancer growth) until it freezes and dies.

These temperature-based treatments have been shown to be extremely effective for a long list of cancers, including skin, breast, and even brain cancer. If you are already undergoing conventional treatment, you may want to speak to your physician about these treatments to see if they can work for your loved one's specific type of cancer and if they can be incorporated into their healing plan, as a wide variety of people have seen great results when using these methods.

Infrared Saunas

As mentioned previously, heat may have an excellent anti-cancer effect when used correctly. For thousands of years, people have enjoyed the health benefits of saunas and steam rooms and the modern incarnation, the infrared sauna, may have even greater health benefits. These types of saunas, as their name so implies, use infrared light at various different wavelengths in order to heat up the body.

Infrared waves penetrate 1 inch into the body, causing toxins, heavy metals, and poisons to be released from our fat and water cells through our sweat. Approximately 20% of this sweat is made up of toxins compared to 2-3% in a conventional sauna.

By heating the body in this manner, you are able to excrete a lot of harmful waste matter from your body through your sweat. Infrared saunas have been shown to get rid of non-essential trace metals such as lead and nickel, as well as being able to inhibit bacterial growth. Even though there is currently not a lot of research that shows that these types of saunas have the ability to directly kill cancer cells, they can help to increase your overall health, vitality, and wellbeing. There are also a host of anecdotal claims from patients saying that infrared sauna use has had positive effects when combined with their cancer treatments.

Infrared saunas can help the body to produce something known as heat-shock proteins. These special little proteins help to make the body more resilient to stress as well as providing a range of other beneficial factors. Therefore, it may be a good idea to ask your doctor if you can add infrared sauna use into your protocol. Please do check though, as some heat therapies are not advised if you are using certain chemo agents due to a skin sensitivity side effect!

Far-infrared saunas are also available to purchase for home use at a reasonable cost.

Near-infared Photoimmunotherapy

Near-infrared photoimmunotherapy is the use of light which uses a united antibody–photoabsorber to bind to cancer cells. When the light is applied, cancer cells have been seen to expand and then burst. Currently, light therapy can only be beneficial where light can reach, limiting the use of cancers that it is able to treat, to skin cancers, and other areas accessible easily by light such as the GI tract.

Ultraviolet Blood Irradiation (UBI)

This therapy is when a small amount of the blood is taken, exposed to UV light, and then reinfused back into the body. This is done as the UV light enhances the biochemical and physiological defences via the blood stream. The process transmits energy into the blood that creates a response in the body and stabilises blood cells. The therapy also increases the venous blood oxygen in patients with lower blood oxygen levels, which helps to eradicate cancer due to the belief that cancer requires an oxygen-free environment to grow. As well as this, UBI is highly anti-inflammatory and enables the body to resist both viral and bacterial infections found in the body.

My Mother's Journey

Unfortunately, due to the chemotherapy tablet that my mum was on, she was unable to continue with the use of heat as a treatment, however, prior to her starting her regimen, we purchased a far-infrared sauna that she was initially using on a daily basis.

****

Chapter Thirteen

Dendritic Cell And Mistletoe Therapy

Dendritic Cell Therapy

Dendritic cell therapy is a personalised vaccine which is made from your own blood.

Dendritic cells are found in your blood. Their job is to identify foreign cells, including cancer cells that may be circulating in your system. Your dendritic cells in a natural state may not be as good as they should be at detecting these cancerous cells. Therefore, dendritic cell therapy as a treatment will retrieve blood from the patient and modify and train the T cells so that they are able to identify cancer cells which they can then kill. They do this by initiating your immune response so that the newly 'trained' cells can be reinjected into the body to boost your body's ability to work against and kill off the cancer.

There have been various positive testimonials from patients who have used this therapy.

Mistletoe Therapy

Mistletoe therapy is one of the most widely studied alternative therapies for cancer with over 2600 published scientific papers. Mistletoe therapy has been shown to stimulate the immune system's response to fight off cancer cells. Mistletoe therapy has been linked to a reduction in tumour growth, and these effects are due to the mistletoe altering the tumour cell biology which can weaken cancer cells, encouraging cancer cell death, which is called apoptosis.

Two of the components of mistletoe - viscotoxins and lectine - have been shown to kill cancer cells in vitro and have been shown to stimulate cancer cells in vitro and in vivo.

Extracts are usually given to patients by injection, however, they can be taken orally or via IV into the pleural cavity or directly into the tumour. Very few side effects have been reported. Many clinical trials have also shown that mistletoe therapy may provide a better quality of life for cancer patients as it reduces several of the side effects associated with chemotherapy and radiation, including cancer-related fatigue.

In Germany, mistletoe injections are approved for use and the treatment is also available in the Netherlands, Switzerland, and the UK, under the names Helixor and Iscador.

****

Chapter Fourteen

Toxins, Chemicals, EMF Exposure,

And Organic Products

Cleansing your body of toxins may be vital for you to achieve optimal health and to beat cancer. Unfortunately, in today's world, these kinds of contaminants are everywhere. It is nearly impossible to escape them. Whether in our food, water supply, clothing, or cutlery, our modern world is bursting at the seams with toxins.

Cancer-causing Toxins

It is widely accepted that everyday substances we are exposed to cause cancer. These substances are also often referred to as carcinogens and unfortunately, their negative effects on the human body go well beyond increasing the risk for cancer. These substances can be found in and around the home in the products that we use for cleaning and general living.

Even though it may seem like an impossible task to completely avoid toxins, there is a lot you can do to benefit your body and to reduce your risk of being exposed to these harmful substances. I have composed a list of a few of the easier steps that you can take to do this:

1.   Use Glass Instead Of Plastics

Even though your wallet may not thank you if you replace everything in your home made of plastic (such as cups and cake trays) with glass, your body certainly will. There are a lot of harmful substances present in plastic and their release can be even greater if it is exposed to heat, such as in the items listed above. One common substance found in plastics that has adverse health effects is BPA. While some companies now pride themselves on creating BPA-free plastics, such as for baby products, others have not bothered to join the revolution. BPA and even some of its replacement counterparts, such as BPS, have been shown to actually aid in the production of cancer cells, as shown in the research of Dr Sumi Dina at the University of Oakland. Using glass instead of plastic will help you to avoid those toxins.

2.   Change Your Cleaning Products

While you may have already thought of this one yourself, let us remind you and give you the facts as to why it is wise to only use a certain type of cleaning product. As a rule of thumb, you want to stay away from products that use bleach as a base, as its fumes can be extremely harmful to our system. When buying your replacements, check the labels and steer clear of anything that includes benzaldehyde and acetaldehyde, as they are both known compounds with carcinogenic effects. It is better to just use ordinary soap or cleaning products that use vinegar as a base.

3.   Filter Your Water

Depending on where you live in the world, a number of different chemicals are being added to your drinking water, which was placed there as an aid against calcification or eutrophication within pipes and water systems. And while these chemicals are good at their respective tasks, they are not so good for your overall health. There are many cheap water filtering products on the market today, however it is best to choose one that removes large amounts of PFAS-based substances (perfluoroalkyl).

As mentioned earlier, saunas and other heat treatments are very good at flushing toxins out of your body. So if you are unable to make these types of lifestyle changes, then it would be good to create a detoxification protocol to assist with your body's ability to deal with these substances.

4.   Change Your Dentist

You may be wondering why this one is on the list. Traditionally, dentists often use heavy metals to treat teeth, such as mercury-based fillings.

It has been scientifically proven that mercury and other heavy metals negatively influence the body, and mercury poisoning is severely dangerous with proven links to cancer. If you have fillings, it is vital that you check what these are made of, as you may have an increased heavy metal overload burdening your immune system, inhibiting your ability to heal. Therefore, either ask your dentist to replace your fillings with healthier alternatives, such as ceramic, or switch entirely to a natural dentist that may have other options available.

Root canals may also be causing your body harm as the procedure carried out by conventional dentists has been known to produce microbes that have been found in patients suffering with breast cancer.

It is therefore advisable to visit your dentist to remove root canals and inquire about a natural holistic dental treatment instead.

Organic Products

In conjunction with the avoidance of certain things, it's a good idea for you to try to make use of as many organic and natural products as possible. Swapping your bleach-based cleaners with the vinegar-based cleaners that were mentioned earlier is a great start. There is also a variety of other products available that you can replace your old products with, that may be more beneficial for your health.

A simple one is to replace your regular food with organic options. While it is more expensive, if you can afford to eat organic produce it is definitely more beneficial to your health.

There are also a variety of natural and organic products on the market that you can use for your personal grooming. Our current shampoos, deodorants and soaps are filled with toxic chemicals that may be harming your system. Natural grooming products are far better for you. Look for personal grooming products with ingredients such as aloe vera, vitamin E, cucumber, coconut oil, and shea butter.

Faith in Nature and Salt of the Earth are recognised brands.

If you are a woman who loves her make–up, you should also know that the vast majority of these products carry harmful toxins that may be detrimental to your health. Fortunately, there are products available, such as CoverFX and BioMineral, who use toxin-free ingredients in their products.

From mascara to nail polish, there are many natural toxin-free alternatives available, most of which can be purchased cost-effectively online.

Heavy Metals

Having touched on the heavy metals used by dentists, I think it's important to cover heavy metals as a whole and include chelation, which is the method of detoxing the body of these metals. Chelating agents are substances that bond with toxins, minerals and metals in your body. Once bonded to them, the chelating agents then carry them out of your body via urine or faeces. Metals such as lead, mercury, and iron can build up in your body over time, which contribute to a toxic load on your system. If you are suffering with a chronic disease or illness, chelation can be used to remove these metals. This should, in turn, help you to heal and repair as it frees up some of the work that your immune system would usually be doing, allowing it to focus on fighting diseases such as cancer.

There is a spray on the market called TRS, which helps your body to detoxify on a cellular level. The spray can be taken daily and will cling to the heavy metal toxins that are circulating in your system via a magnet-like attraction. They will then assist your cells in extracting them out of your body, mainly via urine. As the particles are so tiny, they do not have to be processed via your kidneys. This method allows for a more gentle form of detoxification.

Dr Rashid Buttar, Director of the Centre for Advanced Medicine & Clinical Research has been very prominent in the media for his alternative beliefs.

Dr Buttar believes that most patients with cancer have high levels of heavy metals present, such as mercury and other toxins. His aim is to clear all of the seven main toxins that can be found in the body that cause chronic illness and disease. The seven main toxins of which he focuses his work on are: heavy metals, persistent organic pollutants, pathogens, food, energetic, psychological and spiritual.

Dr Buttar's clinic offers over 50 different IV therapies that assist with the body's detoxification process. His therapies also focus on boosting the immune system in order to help your body to fight the disease.

WiFi Signals – EMF

The EMF (electromagnetic fields) emitted from our phones or cellular masts are known to cause invisible frequencies to disrupt our normal cell functions. The disruption caused by this effectively stops our body's ability to self-repair as it should, which can cause cancer to form. Some studies have shown that long-term mobile phone use has led to double the amount of brain tumours being found in people who use their phones for longer than half an hour every day over several years. In order to try to avoid some of this cellular disruption, it's advised that you turn your phone and WiFi router off when the internet is not in use, avoid keeping the phone too close to the body, take supplements that reduce oxidative stress, use EMF deflective paint in your home if you can, and buy an EMF shield that you can now place on your phones, tablets, and laptops that can protect you from harmful radiation.

You can also hire consultancy companies to do a report with recommendations for your home.

The Verdict

EVERYTHING that we use and consume is processed through our skin and body, and can cause a toxic load build-up.

Toxins can be found pretty much anywhere and everywhere in today's society. There can be toxicity from the plastic that we use to the metals that we use in our frying pans, the wine that we drink and the oils that we cook with. This is why it's best to use organic products and to try to live in a way that is as toxin and BPA-free and friendly as possible.

The benefits of reducing your body's toxic load is that it will allow your body to repair and heal, and get back to its natural state. All of the energy that was being used by your body to kill toxins and detoxify your system will then be freed up to help your body to work as it should. Your body, once in a restorative state, will then use the energy saved in a more productive way, to fight off disease and inflammation.

My Mother's Journey

My mum now only drinks spring mineral water, uses glass as her Tupperware choice, and no longer uses plastics. She uses organic body wash and toxin-free make-up. As a treat, sometimes she will use normal nail varnish, but there are toxin-free nail polishes available.

My mum had her teeth checked by a natural dentist to ensure there are no heavy metals in her dental work.

****

Chapter Fifteen

Intermittent Fasting

Intermittent fasting is a form of fasting that can be practiced every day and in various ways. In its most basic form, it consists of spending a minimum of 12 hours out of a 24 hour period without eating anything and consuming only water. The intermittent fasting protocol can vary, as mentioned, and some practice a 12hour/12hour split while others prefer a 16hour/8hour. A more extreme regimen could consist of consuming only 1 big meal within a 24 hour period. Some say that intermittent fasting can spread to as long as not eating for a period of 48 hours straight, however, this is debated as it is beginning to enter the realm of normal fasting regimens (which have slightly different health benefits). Intermittent fasting is also known as time-restricted-feeding or TRF.

This type of fasting has already been clinically proven to have a variety of effects. These include, but are not limited to: burning body fat while maintaining muscle mass, regulating hormones, balancing blood sugar levels, and increasing insulin sensitivity. The last two aspects can be very beneficial for someone living with diabetes.

Intermittent fasting has been proven to have positive effects on cancer cells. As mentioned earlier, it is highly likely that tumours prefer a high glucose environment in order to thrive as it is their primary source of fuel. It has therefore been theorised that intermittent fasting, due to its ability to drain glycogen stores, has the ability to make cancer cells more vulnerable to attack from immune cells as well as conventional cancer treatments. Fasting has also been proven to induce something known as autophagy, and while this subject could warrant a whole book by itself, we will give you just the brief outline to help you understand. Autophagy is the process by which your body recycles itself. In particular, it breaks down old, dying, and damaged cells, and uses them for spare parts to strengthen your healthy cells. According to research, autophagy has been shown to stop cancer cells from surviving and inducing apoptosis within them by suppressing something known as tumorigenesis.

Intermittent fasting also has positive benefits for the immune system. A large amount of your immune system is interconnected with your gut. In fact, it has been shown that the microbiome, the bacteria that live in your stomach, are so vital for your immune system that some people with immune disorders need a faecal transplant (that is the poop from another person being placed within their stomach) in order for them to regain their gut bacteria and recover their immune system. Intermittent fasting can help to replenish the stem cells within your gut, keeping the lining and walls healthy and strong. This makes sense as your gut lining and walls are unable to adequately repair if they are constantly digesting food. This positive effect on the stomach and your immune system has a variety of anti-cancer benefits, such as activating those T cells that want to kill your cancer.

If you have already begun conventional treatment, intermittent fasting may be a great option for you. Some of the methods we have outlined in this book cannot be used in conjunction with one another, but intermittent fasting is different. In fact, it has been shown, at least in rodent models, that intermittent fasting when used in conjunction with chemotherapy has the ability to not only increase the likelihood of survival but also has the ability to decrease metastasis (secondary tumour growth) and decrease toxicity induced by the treatment. Other animal studies have shown very similar effects on cancer, even when used without conventional treatment.

It may be really beneficial for you or your loved one to begin incorporating an intermittent fasting routine into the protocol. If you are not used to it, you can begin with a 12-hour eating window and, over time, decrease the time within which you eat until you hit your optimal spot. Longer periods are generally better for the effects described, but if you are not used to fasting it may be better to stick to shorter fasting periods, as there is a slight stress response when undergoing intermittent fasting. Once again, make sure to speak to your healthcare provider about any changes you wish to take.

****

Chapter Sixteen

Diet For Cancer Patients

Everything that we consume affects our body's ability to function.

When looking at cancer treatments and therapies it's very easy to forget that, without a good diet and healthy drinking habits, our bodies will struggle to fight disease. As mentioned, there are various treatment options available that can help our body to fight the disease or attack it directly, but we must remember that if our body does not have the necessary nutrients to sustain itself at a healthy level, it will not have the power or energy to survive what we put it through.

In this chapter, we will look at the most researched and popular diets for cancer patients. At the University of Michigan Rogel Cancer Center, Suzzana Zick N.D MPH, one of the members, conducted a study based on comprehensive research on the most popular five diets for cancer patients and these were the findings:

The Alkaline Diet

This diet's philosophy, explained by Zick, is that having an acidic environment in the body causes cancer. Based on this theory, the western diet contains too many animal fats and refined carbohydrates such as pork, red meat, and white flour. Therefore, if someone eats more fruit and vegetables and limits the use of red meat, flour, rice, and sugar, there will be more alkaline ions available for the body after digestion. This extra alkalinity starts decreasing the acid in the body and reduces the strain on the systems in charge of acid-detox, she says.

She then continues by saying: 'You need to eat about 80 percent alkaline foods, like fruit, vegetables, whole grains, and beans, according to this diet.

There is very limited data that the acid nature of your body causes cancer, but by increasing fruit, vegetables and whole grains, and by limiting red meat and simple carbohydrates, you're essentially following the American Cancer Society and WCRF/AICR guidelines and eating foods that decrease cancer mortality and recurrence.'

The Paleo Diet

This diet tries to replicate the Stone Age's dietary pattern of humans. The gatherers and hunters used to eat fruit, vegetables, meat, nuts, and eggs. They also excluded legumes, grains, dairy products, and processed foods. The most devoted followers of the diet believe that chronic illnesses arise from the consumption of foods that came after the agricultural revolution. This is based on the claim that humans are not equipped to digest these foods.

This diet seems to be based on the belief that our ancestors were superior in their eating habits. Zick says that strict adherence to this diet eliminates beans and whole grains, proven to be very beneficial for the prevention of cancer, decreasing cancer mortality, and for health in general. Looking into anthropological evidence, Zick discovered that there seems to be no evidence of a single Palaeolithic diet and that grains used to be processed and consumed even back then. Even though the diet emphasises whole foods, fruits, and vegetables, its followers seem to eat too much red meat.

The Ketogenic Diet

This diet is based on a low-carbohydrate, medium-protein, and high-fat meal plan, with 65% or more of the calories coming from fat. On the Keto diet, the reduction in carbohydrates places your body into a metabolic state which is called ketosis. Once your body is in a ketogenic state, the fat from your body is then burned and used as energy. The diet works to shift cancer's source of energy from glucose to ketones. According to Zick, the research on this is split. Zick says that while half of the evidence is great, the diet itself doesn't contain fruit and vegetables, putting the body in a nutrient deficit which might cause more damage than good.

Zick concludes that cancer cells can find their energy source from ketones as well as glucose, however advocates a healthy eating plan.

Zick's opinion is contradicted by Dr Thomas Seyfried, a biochemical geneticist and professor of biology at Boston College, who believes that cancer can be best defined as a mitochondrial metabolic disease rather than as a genetic disease (which is what many oncologists believe). Otto Warburg originally flagged this in the early 1900s, and Dr Thomas Seyfried, the author of Cancer as a Metabolic Disease, researched this, proving truth behind Otto Warburg's work.

In his book, Dr Thomas Seyfried highlights research that shows cancer is metabolic and not genetic, and it's created when the mitochondria in the body fails (due to the cell's respiration being damaged) which will lead to cancer cells being fed by glutamine and glucose. Dr Seyfried believes that, by placing the body in a ketogenic state and by reducing calories, it places the body in a low blood sugar and elevated ketones state, which will change the source that feeds the cancer, as mentioned above, which can reduce tumours. Several patients that have followed this diet have shown this.

Dr Seyfried recommends that, along with following this diet, his patients should also engage in metabolic therapy through testing, which can highlight any imbalances in the body. This is all done while also undergoing hyperbaric oxygen treatment.

The Vegan Diet

This diet is focused on abstinence from animal products, such as meat, dairy products, eggs, fish, and honey. It also encourages the so-called cancer-fighting foods, like greens, berries, nuts, whole grains, and seeds. An analysis of some vegan studies found that about 15% of cancer patients doing this diet showed improvement in the disease, but they were also exercising, undertaking stress-reducing activity, and most had a good support network.

It was concluded that the results shown could not be completely accurate as the cancer patients were advised to only use this diet with a nutritionist's help in order to ensure that important minerals and nutrients were not missed.

The Macrobiotic Diet

This diet aims to combat the imbalances in the body that cause cancer, and focuses on providing the body with all of the necessary nutrients that it needs. This diet is predominantly vegetarian, however it does also allow unprocessed, organic, and whole foods. Cereal grains, such as rice and millet, make up about 40 to 60% of the diet and the rest is made up of vegetables and legumes. It's high in fibre and free from red and processed meat. This diet was found to increase fibre intake and have a bigger number of micronutrients than the normal daily recommendations. Overall, Zick found it to be a good diet however incomplete, as the results found deficiencies in the normal recommended intake of vitamin D, vitamin B, and calcium.

Zick's Results

Looking at each individual diet, we can see certain benefits from each of them. Zick's findings report that balance is key in a cancer diet. Organic fruit and vegetables, whole foods, and organic white meat, as well as nuts and seeds, with as many greens as possible, will definitely create the balance that the body needs to fight the disease and recover.

It's important to take extra care to avoid processed food and too much sugar. A nutritionist would agree that a healthy diet which gives the body the nutrients that it needs daily is necessary for cancer patients.

I also would like to add a list of cancer-fighting foods that you could try:

» Berries;
» Grapes;
» Tomatoes;
» Whole grains;
» Flaxseeds;
» Broccoli;
» Kale;
» Cabbage and dark-green leafy vegetables; and
» Legumes.

Dr Sebi Diet

Dr Sebi, real name Alfredo Bowman, was a world famous herbalist, natural healer, and tricellular therapist. His belief was that mucus build-up, formed by foods created by an acidic diet, leads to the development of diseases. His theory was that if you create an alkaline environment in your body, disease will not have the ability to survive. His diet and food plans involve focusing on natural, plant-based, alkaline herbs and foods. The Dr Sebi diet encourages people to stay away from acidic and hybrid foods, as they cause harm to the cells in your body.

Dr Sebi created his own nutritional guide, which can be found at www.drsebicellfood.com. Followers of his diet are reminded to drink 1gal of spring water daily, sleep during healing hours 10pm-2am, no longer use the microwave, and avoid any foods and drinks that are not shown on his list. It is also recommended that you avoid canned and seedless fruits, animal products, meat, fish, dairy, honey, GMOs, and all processed sugar and alcohol.

Organic Food And Avoidance Of GMOs

As discussed earlier in the book, it is important to try to eat as organically as possible, and to try to not use genetically modified products when possible. This is due to the many toxins present in these foods. If you are unable to eat organic foods, you should try to wash your fruit and vegetables with 1 tablespoon of vinegar to 1 bowl of water, which will help to remove some of the pesticides present on the products. Alternatively, you can wash them in lemon juice or soak them in ozonated water.

Dairy Products

Some of the world's leading oncologists and cancer experts have publicly discussed the link between dairy and cancer. Milk alone contains nearly 40 different hormones and growth factors that, when studied, shows that the growth stimulant prevents apoptosis - programmed cancer cell death. Milk is sold predominantly in a processed form and goes through a process called pasteurisation, which effectively boils the majority of the goodness out of the milk. Another thing to consider is the high levels of somatic cells found in milk (that is pus cells) which is sold in the supermarket milk that many of us have consumed. The same goes for cheese. It may be a wise idea to think of the above information before purchasing your dairy produce in the future, as it may be hindering yours or your loved ones healing journey.

My Mother's Journey

Diet: My sister really agrees with Dr Sebi's theory, so she printed off a list of foods that my mum should be eating (however, we did alter it slightly to add some more variety).

Please remember that if you are like my mum and are breaking into healthy eating after years of bad habits, you do not have to follow something 100% initially if it doesn't feel right, or your mental health will suffer. Remember that you are allowed to break yourself in to what will become your new way of life. Do not feel bad or judge yourself as this is a new journey for you, so be kind to yourself.

Steroids And Diet:

My mum removed all processed foods, alcohol, and most meats from her diet, although this goes out of the window when she loses her appetite due to her medication that she is on.

▶

When she loses her appetite, she loses weight rapidly and is asked to take steroids to gain some weight - at which point she eats whatever she fancies although, personally, she is still quite restricted.

My mum was doing so well for a year or so, but the weight loss became drastic. (You may or may not be aware that the majority of cancer patients die of malnutrition rather than the cancer itself.) Thus, you have to make your decisions with some caution and logic.

My mum sometimes wants a break from the very strict diet that she is on, so allows herself periods of eating what she fancies as opposed to what her body really needs, which is fine as mental health is an important factor in healing and recovery.

****

Chapter Seventeen

Teas For Cancer Patients

Probably the easiest thing to add into your daily routine is the consumption of tea at regular intervals. Below are the most popular teas that have been shown to have cancer fighting properties:

Green Tea

Green tea is often advertised as a cancer preventive, and this is due to the compound polyphenols which can be found in the tea that is linked to anti-tumour activity. The polyphenols found in green tea can influence the body's system epigenetically (epigenetics is the change in the expressions of genes that has not arisen due to the body's own DNA sequence).

There are various studies that show that green tea helps to boost the immune system. As well as keeping you hydrated, green tea can improve your energy levels. While many studies have been made to prove its cancer prevention abilities, there is not enough information yet to be considered sufficient. However the benefits of green tea should not be ignored. Please keep in mind that green tea usually contains caffeine. If your green tea is decaffeinated via a natural water process, 95% of the antioxidants will be retained, so decaffeinated green tea is always an option if you are trying to avoid caffeine.

Oolong Tea

A 2019 study on Oolong tea extract showed positive results when applied to breast cancer. The effects of the tea, once consumed, showed noticeable damage to the cancer cells. Due to the findings from this research, it may beneficial for you to add Oolong tea to your shopping list when considering drinking teas to fight cancer.

Essiac Tea

This tea is known as one of the most controversial alternative treatments for cancer, and the tea itself contains a few different plants: burdock root, turkey rhubarb root, sheep sorrel, and slippery elm. This tea is sold as a cure for cancer and it has a controversial backstory that makes its reputation untrustworthy for medical professionals. However, it continues to be popular amongst cancer patients and that itself can be a good reason to try it.

JFK's personal doctor tested Essiac and concluded that it does fight cancer cells.

Pau D'Arco

This tea comes from a tree that has several compounds present within its inner bark, mainly lapachol and beta-lapachone, which are thought to be responsible for its health benefits. The properties in this tea have shown to increase macrophage, which helps to fight off cancer cells and increase your immune system's ability to fight off disease.

Pau D'Arco is a natural immune system booster and has been shown to be extremely effective at healing the body, helping it to fight off various other infections present within the body. This tea can be taken in a tincture form or easiest via a tea, and can be purchased from various herbalists and online stores.

Ginger Root Tea

Nausea is one of the most known side effects of chemotherapy. A great anti-nausea remedy is a cup of ginger tea. This tea can be easily made by slicing the ginger root and pouring hot water over it, then allowing it to steep. It would be best to make the tea yourself and avoid purchasing it from the store, but if you choose to do so, then make sure to read the description as some ginger tea is combined with black tea leaves which are not recommended to use alongside certain chemotherapy treatments.

Matcha Green Tea

This is a powdered green tea that is known for its antioxidant properties and a detox agent. Certain studies have shown this tea to have anti-cancer properties. Not only is it high in polyphenols but it is also high in ECGC which is known to reduce inflammation and prevent certain chronic illnesses.

Dandelion Tea

Dandelion tea also has great antioxidant benefits and has been reported as a good digestive aid. In test tubes, dandelion tea has been confirmed as effective to kill cancer cells through lab tests.

My Mother's Journey

My mum has several of the listed teas daily, including Essiac tea and Oolong tea.

****

Chapter Eighteen

Additional Supplements For Cancer Patients

After looking at the importance of a good diet in the fight against cancer and the many benefits that some teas have on cancer, it's important to also cover some of the supplements that are available.

These are some of the most popular cancer-fighting and preventative supplements:

Garlic

Garlic is well-known for its anti-inflammatory effects. Studies have shown that the intake of garlic can inhibit the growth of cancer cells. In 1958, a paper published by Weisberger and Penksy showed that the garlic intake in mice was strongly associated with a reduced risk of gastric, intestinal, and other cancers.

Curcumin

Curcumin, also known as turmeric, is a polyphenol which is a micronutrient that is packed full of antioxidants usually found in plant-based foods. They have been proven to boost digestion, neurofunction, and protect against diabetes and heart disease.

When using curcumin in the fight against cancer, it has been shown to fight cancer at the source, its stem cells, with thousands of reports published and backed by the FDA proving its cancer fighting properties.

Choosing to take an extract of curcumin is the better option, as powders and spices contain as little of 3% of curcuminoids, whereas extracts contain up to 95%.

It has been advised, if new to taking this spice, that you start your dose at 500mg daily. Some cancer patients have been advised to slowly increase their intake to up to 8g daily.

When taking your curcumin extract, try to buy the supplement combined with black pepper, as it increases the effectiveness by up to 1000%.

Studies show that by consuming curcumin daily, you can eliminate 1/3 of human disease.

Make sure to speak to your alternative therapist prior to commencing any new regimen.

AHCC

This is an extract from the mycelia of several species of basidiomycete mushrooms, and it has been shown in studies to reduce the adverse reactions of chemotherapy for cancer patients, especially for advanced cancers.

In a study, people with a history of liver cancer had a higher survival rate when given AHCC compared to the rest of the people in the study. A second study confirmed the first one, where the patients given AHCC had an increased survival rate compared to the ones who were given placebo. Side effects are uncommon but can include diarrhoea and itchiness.

The original patent for AHCC expired so various other companies started to manufacture this. If you wish to add this into your protocol, it's advisable that you try to purchase it from the original Japanese company that conducted all of the studies on this as you are more likely to receive a higher quality product. Alternatively, you can find out the exact ingredients and compare it with their counterparts to ensure you are getting the product and dosage that the original research was based upon.

ALC

This is an amino acid produced in the body, sold as a supplement. This supplement is used mainly to reduce nerve pain from neuropathy. Its effectiveness has been proven in multiple studies, so if you experience nerve pain because of your cancer treatment, this one is definitely worth looking into.

GcMAF

This is a protein produced by the modification of vitamin D-binding protein. GcMAF works in the body by initiating 11 neurological and cellular functions and is known for activating macrophages, the specialised cells that come from white blood cells which contribute to the detection and destruction of harmful organisms and bacteria, such as cancer cells.

It is recommended that, if using GcMAF, it is used alongside other therapies that stimulate the immune system such as therapies that oxidise the body. These bioidentical products can be found on the internet for purchase.

Laetrile, B-17, And Bitter Apricot Kernel

Amygdalin is a compound found in the pit or seeds of various fruits, including bitter apricot kernels. In 1982, a publication deemed amygdalin as a toxic drug that is not effective at fighting cancer, however, various studies since then have demonstrated that this is not the case. Amygdalin has been shown to have major cancer benefits as, during the chemical reactions that take place within the body, amygdalin once broken down creates hydrogen cyanide which can kill cancer cells. People take it in the form of a handful of bitter apricot kernels daily and many have reported great results of their cancer remaining suppressed. The main issues surrounding this is if taken at high doses, the breakdown of amygdalin into hydrogen cyanide can cause serious side effects and poisoning.

Laetrile is a manmade form of amygdalin. Various alternative and integrated cancer clinics will prescribe this to be taken via a drip used in a programme alongside various other supplementation and vitamin therapy.

Research has shown mixed results, and there have been no controlled clinical trials to date.

Astragalas

This supplement is popular in Chinese herbal medicines. Traditionally, it is used as a tonic to treat tiredness, anaemia, shortness of breath, and other conditions. It is also used to enhance the immune system. Its effects are also anti-inflammatory, antioxidant, and anti-cancer.

Recent studies have shown that *astragalus membranaceus* (AM) and *angelica sinensis* (AS) can benefit patients with lung cancer and cachexia. Cachexia is a complex issue also known as wasting syndrome which consists of the cancer patient experiencing conditions similar to anorexia, weight loss, anaemia, and asthenia. Scientists are still unsure as to what triggers cachexia but they do know that it affects various organs within the body at once. The combination of *astragalus membranaceus* (AM) and *angelica sinensis* (AS) therapy has been proven to have anti-cancer and anti-cachectic effects.

BEC

This is a mix of compounds known as solasodine rhamnosides. They are extracted from the devil's apple fruit and from the eggplant. It is mostly used as a topical cream for skin cancer patients.

Boswellia Serrata

This is an extract from a tree with the same name and is popular in Ayurvedic medicine. Also known as Indian frankincense, it is used in the West as an anti-inflammatory. Frankincense appears to be fairly non-toxic and is commonly prescribed by integrated cancer specialists in oil form for inhalation or topical use. Patients that have brain cancer or metastases to the brain have been known to use the oil in a diffuser as it has been shown to reduce swelling. Various studies have shown that frankincense may have the ability to target cancer cells without killing healthy cells.

These supplements each have their own benefits and side effects. It is therefore important to discuss them with either your therapist or a nutritionist before taking them, as they can have an effect on your current treatment plan.

Feverfew

Feverfew is a flowering plant that comes from the family of daisies, commonly used to prevent migraines and headaches. Feverfew has a compound called parthenolide, which has been found to block the formation of inflammatory proteins. Various animal lab studies have shown that Feverfew also shows anti-cancer effects, however, human studies are required to verify this. With various herbs, the positive properties can be extracted into a tincture with 100% alcohol and ingested. Once you have taken the dose in tincture form, the compounds will go directly into the bloodstream at maximum dose. If the extract is made into a capsule, the extract will go through the digestive process and will be absorbed into the body in a different way, and may lose some of its anti-cancer properties. Some cancer patients may choose to make a tea with the extract.

Nitric Oxide

John Hewlett has designed a supplement called Cardio Miracle which is a nitric oxide supplement. Nitric oxide aids proper cellular function and is critical in the human cell replication process. Nitric oxide supports the body during the detoxification process while helping to maintain a healthy body.

John Hewlett advocates the use of vitamin D with nitric oxide, as vitamin D extends the life of nitric oxide within the body. Nitric oxide is used in order to protect against the development and progression of cancer.

Low levels of vitamin D is linked to colorectal cancer, bladder and bowel cancer, along with various other cancers such as breast cancer.

Haelan

Haelan is a formula that was developed in order to provide nutritional support for patients recovering from chemotherapy or other treatments. It contains 25lbs of soy (organic and non GMO). Soy contains isoflavones and genistein. Genistein, in high concentrations, has been shown to induce breast cancer cell death as well as helping to enhance the effects of radiation in various breast cancer cells and other cancer cells including pancreatic cancer.

Bicarbonate Of Soda

Bicarbonate of soda is one of the most cost effective ways to balance your body's PH levels and to alkalise the body. There are several clinics that offer bicarbonate therapy, but if money is tight, you can opt for purchasing an aluminium-free brand and adding some to your water, juices, smoothies, enemas, or your bath. Dr Mark Sircus has a book called Sodium Bicarbonate - Rich Man's Poor Man's Cancer Treatment that can assist you with your bicarb protocol.

My Mother's Journey

Supplements:

My mum had a consultation with an integrated cancer specialist who advised her to take several supplements to enhance her health. I would recommend speaking to one when you can in order to get a tailored list of supplements that are specific to your needs.

Bitter Kernels:

My mum has a handful of these nuts daily.

Astragalas:

My mum has been diagnosed with cachexia and was recommended various supplements to help her to gain weight. At this point, she had completely lost her appetite, was feeling sick a lot of the time, and was constantly exhausted. She then started on astragalas, which seems to have improved her appetite and fatigue.

▶

Frankincense (Boswellia Serrata) :

Upon diagnosis of brain metastases, my aunt purchased frankincense that my mum started to use in a diffuser in order to inhale the oil.

Garlic And Turmeric (Curcumin):

My mum takes a daily dose of garlic and turmeric in capsule form. (My mum does not react well to the capsule itself so she removes the outer shell of the capsule and adds the contents of the capsule into a liquid, which she will then swallow).

****

Chapter Nineteen

CBD, Hemp, And THC

Cannabis has been scientifically proven to have a great range of medicinal benefits associated with the compounds found in the plant. The two major components of this plant are known as THC, or tetrahydrocannabinol, and CBD, or cannabidiol. These two compounds have profound effects when ingested into the human body because of a system that each and every one of us carries: the endocannabinoid system.

Endocannabinoid System

The ECS is a system that is found throughout our body whose primary function is to maintain homeostasis. We are constantly exposed to different external stressors, such as heat, cold, toxins, radiation, jobs, our children, etc. When these things are starting to cause too much of a negative impact, then the endocannabinoid system helps to maintain neuroplasticity, which can alleviate anxiety and depression (both common symptoms of becoming overly stressed). Chronic inflammation is also something that the ECS handles. It does this by balancing processes that produce and regulate inflammation within the body, making you feel weak or ill. This is via its impact on the immune system. But how does the ECS work, specifically?

The ECS is spread out within your body and is made up out of a large network of receptor sites and molecules for signalling. Don't worry if this sounds a bit technical, there are actually only a few things you need to know. There are two types of receptor sites known as CB1 and CB2 receptors. Whenever the stress levels in your life increase, the body releases the signalling molecules, the endocannabinoids, to go and bind to your CB1 and CB2 receptors. Through this process, many other signals are sent throughout the body which helps to balance systems and stabilise responses. ECBs are naturally produced by the body, but can be impaired through improper diet and a lack of regular exercise, as well as other lifestyle choices. If none of these are monitored properly, then the system cannot function the way it was designed to.

As mentioned earlier, one of the primary ways in which your ECS interacts with your body is via its connection to the immune system. In fact, immune cells are covered in CB2 receptor sites designed for your ECBs. The main types of endocannabinoids that your body releases are called anandamide and 2-AG. When they connect to the receptors located on the immune cell, they help to reinitialise calming after a strong immune response, decreasing inflammation. The balance between inflammation and lack thereof is extremely important to maintaining health. However, as mentioned before, several things can disrupt the partnership between these two systems, and this is where CBD can potentially come to the rescue.

CBD And THC For Cancer

As you have already seen, the endocannabinoid system has various beneficial effects on the body. By using its ability to help to maintain a proper function of the immune system, it aids in releasing T cells which destroy cancer cells. CBD specifically has the ability to induce a lot of the same effects that your endogenous cannabinoids have, thereby strengthening the immune system.

There is also a lot of clinical research going into CBD and its direct effect on cancer. It has been proven in a laboratory setting that CBD has the ability to cause the death of cancer cells, block their growth, and inhibit the development of blood vessels which are necessary for cancers to grow. While more research is required within human study participants, this is excellent news for anyone who is afflicted with cancer. CBD has recently undergone a large cultural shift, which means that its research is now being funded to greater degrees, and wellness products containing CBD are readily available on the market.

You do not have to smoke it to ingest it. There are a variety of different ways you can take CBD. Some of the easiest would be gummies that have been infused with the compound or oils which can be dripped into the mouth using a pipette. Most CBD wellness products are known as full-spectrum products. This means that they also contain trace amounts of other cannabinoids as well as THC. Keep this in mind if you want a CBD-only product and remember to ask your doctor for advice when adding anything new into your protocol.

CBD And Hemp Oil

Hemp and marijuana are both varieties of the sativa plant. Both contain CBD and THC, which are the two most active ingredients.

Hemp has much less THC than a typical marijuana plant, so it is less likely to cause hallucinations and lethargy.

Some cancer sufferers have testified that hemp and/or CBD oil has caused their side effects from conventional treatments to reduce, while some have cited that it has even caused their cancer to regress.

If you are interested in taking CBD or hemp oil, it's best to speak to your alternative or integrated cancer specialist in order to obtain the correct dosage that you should be taking.

Rick Simpson Oil

Rick Simpson Oil (RSO), which is also known as Phoenix Tears, is a type of super-concentrated cannabis extract developed by Rick Simpson. Cannabis extract may not be a new thing, but the focus on high dosages of concentrated THC makes RSO unique. The oil produced by Rick Simpson's method advocates the use of the bud from indica strains of cannabis only, as it produces a calming effect that allows the body to heal.

THC has been shown to help to control various side effects of chemotherapy. Several studies have shown that THC has stopped the growth of tumours in relation to lung, breast, skin, and other cancers, while sparing healthy cells. This comes alongside all of its other health benefits, such as treating diabetes, heart disease, and chronic pain.

You will find testimonies all over the internet of cancer patients saying that they have cured their cancer using this oil. The downside to this oil, however, is that THC has strong psychoactive effects. Due to the high levels of THC in this oil, it is illegal to buy in many countries but if you are in the USA or Canada and you live in a state that has legalised marijuana, you may be able to purchase it from a cannabis dispensary.

The RSO method for cancer is to build up to ingesting 60ml of pure THC oil over a 90 day period. There are several testimonies of people that have managed this dose, or near, and have seen a regression or suppression of their cancer growth.

Should you be in a country where cannabis is legal and are interested in making it yourself, you can easily do so with instructions found on the internet. One website is https://www.wikihow.com/Make-Rick-Simpson-Oil.

CBD Oil To THC Ratio

It is recommended that when taking THC, you also take a high strength CBD oil to supplement this. Please look into the RSO method further to see the exact recommended dosage.

Suppositories

Some patients who are unable to reach the desired RSO dosage due to the side effects of taking it orally may prefer to make suppositories for insertion into the rectum.

Several cancer sufferers who have tried this method say that they find that the THC is not as effective rectally as it gets broken down via the digestive tract which dilutes the potency. Several other sufferers who use RSO have suggested trying to get the THC as close to the cancer source as possible in order to gain maximum effect, i.e. if you had cancer of the throat, collar, arm, etc., consuming it rectally would not be the best option.

If you choose the RSO route, please ensure that you carry out adequate research to ensure that your dosage and method is correct and will be beneficial to you. Also be prepared to rest and sleep a lot, which will help your body to heal.

Paediatric Cancer And CBD/THC

If you are looking for guidance on paediatric cancer, you must seek advice from professionals that provide specialist advice in this field.

I am aware of various stories where medical cannabis has been used by parents whose children have paediatric cancer.

Cannakids is a company that was set up by a mother whose daughter was diagnosed with cancer and provides products and services that can assist you further on paediatric cancer treatments. Please do not start any treatments without consulting a paediatric specialist or healthcare provider.

My Mother's Journey

RSO - THC/Cannabis Oil:

When my mum initially started THC, she was unable to take the side effects associated with the oil, however, she persevered regardless. We found a story online of a lady who had been diagnosed with the same cancer as my mum and had the same problem of struggling to manage the side effects of the THC when taking it orally. In the story, the lady's husband discovered that you could take RSO as a suppository via the rectum in order to bypass the side effects, so he went about making these for his wife. After the 90 days were up, tests showed that she had gone into complete remission.

Due to this story, my mum decided that it was worth trying the suppository method, so my mum started taking 1ml of THC in suppository form daily.

Once my mum built up tolerance to the THC, she started introducing it back orally.

▶

While using the RSO method, you are encouraged to use CBD oil alongside the THC. My mum supplemented her THC intake with extra strength CBD oil at 1ml per CBD per 1ml of THC .

My mum had to build up her tolerance to the RSO so started to take the recommended half a rice grain size every day to start with. Remember that if you cannot tolerate the dose, reduce it to a dose that you can manage.

There are several side effects side effects associated with RSO so make sure to do your research before commencing this therapy.

****

Chapter Twenty

Repurposed Drugs

Repurposed drugs are drugs that were originally created for other medical conditions but are now being turned to by alternative and integrated health practitioners for the treatment of cancer. Some of the repurposed drugs available include anti-parasitic drugs, antibiotics, and cold and flu treatments, with many people testifying that the use of these drugs have helped them in their fight with cancer and, in some cases, helped them to beat their disease.

A simple internet search of 'cancer cures through repurposed drugs' will bring up various stories similar to the above.

A story that springs to mind is of a man in the USA who cured his cancer though the use of fenbendazole - a dog dewormer. The brand he used was Panacur Canine Dewormer, which contained 222 mg of fenbendazole. As well as using the fenbendazole, he also was taking 600mg of curcumin in the form of 2 pills per day and 25mg of CBD oil under the tongue each day.

I have listed the names of some of the repurposed drugs that I have encountered during my research on this journey that have been linked to cancer treatments:

» Fenbendazole - an anti-parasite drug that has been shown to have significant anti-cancer benefits.
» Mebendazole is similar to fenbendazole and has shown promise in the fight against cancer.
» Antihistamines - antihistamines have been used to reduce the spread of cancer and increase survival rates.

» Metformin - metformin, used for diabetes, has been shown to have anti-cancer benefits and cancer cell killing abilities, as well as being an being an anti-inflammatory compound.

» Low Dose Naltrexone (LDN) has been shown to stabilise some prostate and colorectal cancers. LDN has also been shown to be effective in treating various other cancers.

These are some of the most common repurposed drugs available. Some of the other drugs used are methadone, chloroquinine, aspirin, and doxycycline, to name a few.

The Care Oncology Clinic, who have a clinic in Harley Street, London, as well as in the USA, specialise in repurposed drugs for cancer patients and offer face-to-face as well as virtual consultations.

The ReDO project are an organisation that can be found online. They have compiled a list on their website with over 270 different drugs that can be repurposed in order to treat cancer patients.

My Mother's Journey

My mum has a friend who was seeing a specialist that prescribed repurposed drugs and had great results at keeping her cancer at bay. It is an option that will be revisited in the future if and when my mum's current medication stops working.

****

Chapter Twenty-One

Extra Tests: Biocept Test, RGCC Test, And Navarro HCG Test

There are various tests that can be undertaken that can assist you in finding out additional information on your cancer. The tests I will cover are the Biocept test and the RGCC test which are a blood tests, and the Navarro test which is a urine test.

Biocept Test

The Biocept test works by obtaining a liquid biopsy (blood sample) from the patient, the sample is sent to the Biocept laboratory in order to look for any biomarkers that can be found in circulating tumour cells. These tests can be used if doctors are unable to obtain a sufficient sample from biopsy, or to gain a better understanding of any metastasising cancer. The results can help your oncologist and therapist to provide the best all-rounded treatment for the specific cancer tested.

If you are trying to monitor the cancer, the Biocept test can also help by keeping track of cancer markers. This will allow you to stay informed on what is happening in yours or your loved ones body, prior to any hospital MRI or CT scans. This may allow you or your loved one to increase any alternative treatments or various supplements and therapies should the markers start to rise, which may contribute to a slower spread or stopping of the disease.

RGCC Test

RGCC tests offer liquid biopsy tests, circulating tumour cell tests, and circulating free DNA tests. These tests are designed to discover any undetected cancer in your system and screen and analyse any cancer cells that may already be present. These tests can be used to monitor existing cancers and provide a personalised plan on which natural treatments and chemotherapy drugs are best suited to your individual genetic makeup.

The RGCC personalised test is effective, as it can help to pinpoint genetic instability and can help to identify where there are imbalances in your own body. The results can then be interpreted to show you what does or does not work well with your body. For example, you can test your chemotherapy drugs against your own genetics to see if they are effective at fighting off cancer in your body. The RGCC onconomics plus test tests 48 various natural substances and anti-cancer drugs to see how they interact with your own cells.

Navarro Test

Developed in the late 1950s by the renowned oncologist, the late Dr Manuel D. Navarro, the test detects the presence of cancer cells even before signs or symptoms develop. Dr Navarro found HCG to be present in all types of cancers. The test is based on a theory proposed by Howard Beard and other researchers who contend that cancer is related to a misplaced trophoblastic cell that becomes malignant in a manner similar to pregnancy, in that they both secrete HCG. As a consequence, a measure of the amount of HCG found in the blood or urine is also a measure of the degree of malignancy. The higher the number, the greater the severity of cancer. Urine, as opposed to blood or serum, is the preferred specimen for the test. In 1980, Papapetrou and co-authors reported the correctness of the urine specimen to be used in HCG immunoassay. In 32 proven cancer cases, the immunoassay test gave 31 positive results using urine while only 12 positive results were reported using blood. HCG has been found to undergo glycosylation in the liver as it travels in the hepatic circulation. Thus, the HCG molecule cannot be detected. The molecule does not undergo this process in the kidney and therefore the molecule remains intact in the urine, which is how the results are obtained.

The test detects the presence of brain cancer as early as 29 months before symptoms appear; 27 months for fibrosarcoma of the abdomen; 24 months for skin cancer; 12 months for cancer of the bones (metastasis from the breast extirpated 2 years earlier).

The Navarro Medical Clinic has been performing the HCG test for cancer for many years and continues to offer this service under the direction of Dr Efren Navarro. Dr Efren Navarro, the son of the late Dr Manuel D Navarro, is a graduate of Doctor of Medicine from the University of Santo Thomas, School of Medicine and Surgery, Manila Philippines. He finished his residency in Pathology at Mercy Hospital Medical Center in Chicago. In 1994, he became a Hematopathology Fellow at the University of Illinois, Chicago. In 1996, he returned to the Philippines to continue the work of his famous oncologist father, Manuel Navarro, M.D.

Currently, many cancer patients take advantage of the diagnostic accuracy of the HCG test as an indicator of the effectiveness of their specific mode of therapy. Thousands of cancer survivors have used this test over the years to keep track of their treatment(s) success and check on the status of their remission. Patients follow a simple direction for preparing a dry extract from the urine sample. The powdery extract is then mailed to the Navarro Medical Clinic in the Philippines, where the HCG testing procedure is then performed*.

HCG Specimen Test Preparation -
details taken from navarromedicalclinic.com

Materials Needed

1. Acetone - can be purchased from the Pharmacy or Hardware or Paint Store. Nail Polish Remover is NOT A SUBSTITUTION unless it is clearly stated in the bottle that it is 100% Acetone;
2. Alcohol - either Ethyl or Isopropyl or Rubbing. The higher the percent of alcohol content, the better to use;

3. Coffee Filter - white or brown;
4. Plastic sandwich bag;
5. Beaker or any glass container or glass jar;
6. Glass measuring cup; and a
7. Measuring spoon.

Preparation Steps

1. From an early morning urine, take 50 ml (1.7 oz) and add 200 ml (7 oz) of acetone and 5 ml (1 teaspoon) of alcohol. Stir and mix well. * Note: 1 ml = 1 cc.
2. Let it stand in the refrigerator or cool place for at least **6 hours** until sediments are formed. Throw off about half of the urine-acetone mixture without losing any sediment. Shake the mixture and filter the remainder through a coffee filter making sure all the sediments are on the filter paper. You may place the filter paper in a glass jar to hold in place prior to filtering.
3. When filtration is over, air dry indoors the filter with its sediments.
4. When dry, fold, wrap it with a sandwich plastic bag.
5. Mail it using the First Class Mail to:

Dr Efren Navarro, MD
3553 Sining Street
Morningside Terrace
Santa Mesa, Manila 1016
Philippines
To see other Mailing Options-
https://www.navarromedicalclinic.com/mailing.php

With the specimen please include a note stating the Patient's Name, Address, Gender, Date of Birth, Email Address, Date when specimen was Created, a brief Clinical History and/or diagnosis.

Copy of the Payment Check or a copy of the receipt of the Western Union or MoneyGram.

The current charge as of October 2020 is $63 US Dollars, payable to Efren Navarro. Mail payments to: Efren Navarro , 820 N. Coolidge Ave, Palatine IL 60067

Please allow 3-4 weeks for test result delivery when mailing from USA, Canada or Europe.

Precautions

Before collecting the urine sample, make sure that there is NO sexual contact for 12 days for Female patients, 48 hours for Male. **DO NOT SEND URINE IF THE PATIENT IS PREGNANT.**

Additional Interferences with the Test:
1. Thyroid hormones.
2. Steroidal compounds (i.e. prednisone).
3. Female hormone supplements (estrogen, testosterone, progesterone).
4. Vitamin D.

If you are using these compounds you must wait for three days after you stop taking them and resume after urine extraction. **AS ALWAYS, CONSULT YOUR PHYSICIAN PRIOR TO STOPPING ANY MEDICATIONS OR SUPPLEMENTS.**

Details taken directly from Navarro Medical Clinic website as authorised by Dr Efren Navarro.

Personalised Tests

There are also several other specific oncological tests available where you can send in samples of blood or biopsies for personalised results to be obtained. The results provided from several of these alternative tests will allow for an individualised cancer treatment plan rather than the one-size-fits-all cancer solution that is given from the majority of western doctors.

My Mother's Journey

While this book was being published, my mum received her results back from the RGCC test that she had taken. The test results for the natural substances that could potentially help her in her journey can be found after the references at the back of this book. A protocol will be put into place which will be added to her current healing plan .

A copy of the other results received can be found at www.ndlondon.co.uk. All of my mum's personal details have been removed and all results shared are oncological test results based on her specific genomes and are shared for information purposes only.

****

Chapter Twenty-Two

Exercise

Various studies have shown that exercise is vital when beating cancer.

Linda Brooks, the author of Rebounding and Your Immune System, advises cancer patients to spend two minutes gently bouncing on a mini trampoline or rebounder every hour. Rebounding has anti-inflammatory effects, as the movement helps to stimulate your lymphatic drainage system, which is the system in your body that helps to rid the body of waste and toxins.

Exercise can specifically improve cancer-related fatigue and can improve survival rates in some cancers.

Studies at the Centre for Active Health in Denmark, published in Cancer Research, concluded that adrenalin released during intensive training prevents metastases and the spread of cancer throughout the body. The study indicated that it may be optimal for women with breast cancer to exercise 2 x per week at a high intensity in order to reduce the spread of the disease. The study showed that exercise can reduce the risk of breast cancer developing by as much as 25 per cent while improving the chances of a successful cancer treatment.

Yoga, tai chi, pilates, or gentle stretches are also great forms of exercise that can be performed if the body is not up to a workout at a higher level. These gentle exercises can allow the mind to focus on the movement and breath, allowing the mind a moment to release from the emotion that accompanies a cancer diagnosis. Maybe encourage your loved one to take a walk with you and then spend some time trying to stretch peacefully after.

There are several clinics worldwide that specialise in exercise rehabilitation after a cancer diagnosis in order to encourage mobility, health, and fitness, as it is vital for the body as a whole.

My Mother's Journey

My mum purchased a rebounder and was using the rebounder for 2 minutes every hour initially. Eventually, it became too much of a task for her to keep up the timings, so instead she aims to use the rebounder every day for at least 10 minutes.

****

Chapter Twenty-Three

Grounding, Emotional Release,

And Mindful Meditation

While we have spent the vast majority of this book focusing on what you can do to ensure that you can have a healthy body and you are prepared to take on the cancer with all the physical tools necessary, it is also extremely important to remember that you are only human. As a human being, there are a variety of different, difficult, and complex emotional and mental factors that need to be considered and addressed when it comes to dealing with cancer. This goes far beyond just the initial shock that comes with such a diagnosis. It is vital for anyone involved to give ongoing care to their mental and emotional wellbeing, as many of us fail to comprehend the strong link between the body and mind.

Stress is a proven contributing factor to the spread of cancer, therefore cellular healing on this level may help to combat the disease.

Grounding And Emotional Release

According to the Eddins Counselling Group, grounding is a particularly beneficial technique as it is a way to self-soothe and deal with difficult emotions and stressful situations. While many who suffer from cancer are blessed enough to have a fantastic support network around them to assist with their needs, the fight against cancer can never be truly separated from the patient. Therefore, learning these techniques, or sharing them with your loved one, would be invaluable in allowing them to continue having a great quality of life.

While grounding may sound very similar to other techniques, such as yoga or meditation, it is slightly different in its methodology and approach .

The primary aspect that differentiates grounding is the fact that it is based on the focus on something within the physical world. It is easy for someone dealing with a stressful situation like cancer to become absorbed in their own thought process. Often, these thoughts can be extremely negative and may cause a bad spiral which can make you feel lost or helpless. Therefore, it is important to learn how to bring your attention away from those thoughts and one of the best ways to do that is by focusing on what is in front of you. Here are some helpful examples that anyone could implement into their everyday routine:

» Turn on a tap and run some cold water across your hands.
» Put an icepack on your forehead for 30 seconds.
» Press the heels of your feet starkly into the ground.
» Clench your fists as tight as you can.
» Describe the flavours of the food you're eating to yourself in your mind.
» The 5, 4, 3, 2, 1 technique – name five things you see, four things you hear, three things you can touch within your reach, two things you smell, and one thing you can taste.

By implementing these grounding techniques, you will gain the ability to take yourself away from your negative thought patterns, should they ever arise, which will empower you to live the kind of life that you want to live despite your situation.

Emotional Release Techniques

This therapy, as the name already suggests, focuses on the dispersal of negative emotions that are a by-product of negative thoughts.

These emotions and thoughts are often created by self-doubt or stressful events, such as being diagnosed with cancer. Emotional release techniques can have an amazing effect on those struggling with these types of emotions.

While there are some different approaches to this technique, one that is well received by patients is the emotional release protocol utilised by the Integrative Wellness Group. For their treatment, they often place patients within small groups of four people, or even less, as this allows for a greater amount of one-on-one attention with the practitioner.

The clinic uses a variety of different methods that allow you to release your pent-up emotional stressors. Some of these include timeline therapy, in which the purpose is to pinpoint exactly where the root cause of your trauma may be, muscle testing, designed to release the subconscious mind of negative emotions, as well as cold laser therapy, which targets the meridian centres found within ancient Chinese medicinal practices. This is great for releasing blockages within your energy system, which should allow your chi to flow naturally.

Stress and negative emotions are very visceral and physical, and therefore often times, as part of emotional release therapy, modern technologies that deal with this problem may be integrated. This includes the use of BioScan SRT, which combines aspects from various disciplines, including biofeedback, acupuncture, and homeopathy. However, if you are not able to attend a clinic such as the one described above, you do not have to worry. There are many other emotional release techniques that you can utilise for free at home. The technique outlined below is based on credible emotional healing practitioner Deepak Chopra.

1. Find yourself a quiet spot in your house where you can be alone for a few moments.
2. Close your eyes and focus on the moment you first experienced the pain of your diagnosis. It may have been in the doctor's office, or it could have been months later during your treatment, but if you have emotional pain associated with this illness then there is a moment in time where that pain was created.

3. Relive that moment as a quiet observer. Try to reimagine it as vividly as you possibly can, without judging it or falling too deeply into the events.

4. Feel the emotion associated with the event; is it fear, anger, hatred? Try and place a name on the pain.

5. Express the feeling by placing it in the real world. Often you will feel the pain somewhere in your body, say out loud where it hurts. If you cry at the pain, that is fine. If you are struggling to express the feeling, you can also write your feelings down.

6. Make the choice that from now on, you will react differently to this stimulus. You will no longer feel as though it is controlling you and you take responsibility for the pain and realise that it is within your power how you react to the pain you feel.

7. Release the painful emotion by focusing again on where in your body it hurts. Really dig into the feeling of the pain and breathe your way through it. After several minutes, the pain should start to dissipate.

8. Tell other people about what you went through if you are able to. Sharing your progress will definitely allow you to grow and heal from your emotional pain more quickly.

Meditation

Meditation is different from grounding because its focal point does not have to be based on sensory input, though it can be. If you are already a practitioner of meditation or have been involved in some way in the wellness community, you may already be aware of how regenerative the practice really is, as meditation and health go hand-in-hand.

Meditation can come in various forms, some of which focus on movements incorporated in tai chi and chi gong. The way that you perform meditation in its most basic form is to recognise that your mind is racing and filled with thoughts. Once you have recognised this state of mind, your aim is to direct your attention to the present moment while focusing on the still in the here and now.

Numerous studies have shown that meditation has a positive effect on those suffering from cancer. If you are undergoing conventional treatment for cancer, there is a chance that you may experience some pain. Many cancer sufferers practice meditation as a non-invasive way to manage their pain, without side effects.

The benefit of meditation does go a lot further than helping with pain relief. Elevated stress levels have long been linked to ill health and if you are suffering from cancer, you will need to do everything you can to decrease your stress levels and the rise in the stress hormone cortisol which, when left unchecked, can damage your body further. Meditation has been shown in clinical trials to be able to reduce the stress amount by a significant margin. Therefore, if you are often feeling stressed about your situation, it would be beneficial to your health if you practiced meditation.

Other studies have shown that meditation can have benefits on various other health factors, including lowering your blood pressure, helping you to fall asleep quicker, and breathe more calmly and deeply. The best thing about meditation is the fact that it is easy to learn and that you can do it for free. However, should you feel the need to find an instructor, there are many available that charge a relatively small fee.

How To Perform Meditation

As mentioned before, there are several different ways to perform meditation, but here is a simple meditation routine you can practice at home without the need for any specialist equipment or teaching.

1. Find a quiet place where you can be alone for several minutes.
2. Sit down and get into a comfortable position. This can be on a chair or on the floor, whichever is easier for you.

3. Start by breathing in and out slowly for a couple of minutes. You can count your breath as you do this, as it will allow you to capture your focus.

4. Continue to focus on your breath as you breathe in and out. It is important to have an anchor point for your meditation (in this case, your breath). Whenever you feel your thoughts drifting and you realise it, bring your attention back to your own breath.

5. Repeat this for about 15 minutes. It may be good to play special music designed for meditation that can be found for free online while you practice.

6. Remember that meditation is a skill and you will not be able to be great at it overnight. Many people have spent years practicing, so just keep trying. If it is hard for you please persevere, as it does become easier with time and the health benefits are worth it.

****

Chapter Twenty-Four

Spirituality

Spirituality can affect various physiological mechanisms, which can positively affect our health.

Hope, contentment, forgiveness, and love are all emotions that are encouraged in many spiritual traditions. This serves us by affecting the neural pathways that connect to the endocrine and immune systems.

Whether you believe in God, Allah, Jah, Jehovah, Buddhist teachings, or you are a believer in any other faith, higher purpose, or power, studies have shown that faith is a powerful force that helps people to achieve an inner sense of calm and wellbeing.

Faith, in this instance, can work by offering you support and guidance about what will happen next. Your faith can be used as a purpose to continue the fight to live. It can help you to embrace feelings of love and kindness while condemning feelings such as anxiety, anger, aggression, resentment, and hostility that can accompany a cancer diagnosis.

Faith can give one hope for the future and acceptance for the things outside of their control.

My Mother's Journey

My mum has kept her Christian faith during her whole cancer journey, and has never questioned God's reasoning for her having cancer. Instead, she tries to focus on healing and remaining as positive as possible at all times.

****

Chapter Twenty-Five

Clinical Trials And

Tests Available For Cancer Patients

Clinical trials are research studies that review how well a new type of treatment can work on people. There are trials that focus on late-stage disease, some focus on preventing cancer, some for improving early diagnosis, for stopping cancer from coming back, or for reducing the side effects of certain treatments for a better quality of life.

Dr David Carbone, from Ohio State University, said: "The treatments we use today were discovered, tested and first made available to patients in clinical trials—and the drugs that are the future of cancer treatment are in trials today. I want to emphasise that being in a clinical trial is how you get access to the next generation of cancer treatment."

There are many available clinical trials out there for cancer patients, and the way you can find them is by going to cancer-specific clinical trial list's and finding a trial based on your specific disease, its type, and stage. These are a few websites that provide access to clinical trials, and you can choose one of them or more to find clinical trials that you may like to participate in.

» BreastCancerTrials.org: This website can help you find a clinical trial for breast cancer if that is your case. It also includes a separate search engine for metastatic breast cancer and you can set it up to notify you when there are new ones available.

» Melanoma Research Alliance (MRA): Their website helps you to find a clinical trial based on your answers to a series of questions.

» Metastatic Breast Cancer Project (MBCproject): This is a project that helps researchers gather information on metastatic breast cancer and that information will be used for new treatment approaches.

» Metastatic Prostate Cancer Project (MPCproject): This project gathers information on metastatic and advanced prostate cancer and the information will be used for studying new treatment options.

» National Brain Tumour Society Clinical Trial Finder: With this database, you are able to search for clinical trials in relation to brain tumours.

» Pancreatic Cancer Action Network Clinical Trial Finder: You are able to find clinical trials in relation to pancreatic cancer with this service.

» SPOHNC Clinical Trial Navigation Service: This resource is available to support people with oral, head, and neck cancer. It allows them to speak to a clinical trial navigator or use the diagnosis tool.

» The Leukemia & Lymphoma Society Clinical Trial Support Center: This particular service was created to support people with leukaemia and lymphoma. With it, people can chat with one another and connect with specialists in the relevant fields.

» Us TOO Prostate Cancer Clinical Trial Finder: If you are looking for a prostate cancer clinical trial finder then this service has you covered. It provides a network for people as well as online support and education.

» You can run a search for clinical trials available for yours or your loved one's specific type of cancer at the below sites:
   » https://www.cancer.gov/about-cancer/treatment/clinical-trials/search if you are in the USA.
   » https://www.cancerresearchuk.org/about-cancer/find-a-clinical-trial if you are in the UK.

» https://www.clinicaltrialsregister.eu/joiningtrial.html if you are in Europe.

SapC-DOPS

This is an innovative new approach to treating lung cancer developed by Dr Xioyang Qi of the University of Cincinnati, who was kind enough to lend me his research for this section. (Please refer to the reference list for further details of his work.) SapC-DOPS is a new type of compound with therapeutic effects. It utilises a nanotechnology drug delivery system known as nanovesicle in order to deliver biomarkers directly to the cancer cell. The therapy shows great promise, because it can target very specific cells without affecting those around it, meaning it can be used to target only cancer cells. SapC-DOPS is a combination of cell protein, SapC, phospholipids, and DROPS, all assembled together in an organised fashion. During his research, he has found that this approach is likely to inhibit tumour growth and potentially increase survival when combined with other therapies. This therapy is currently in the clinical trial stages.

****

Chapter Twenty-Six

Cancer Therapies On A Budget

If money is not in abundance, you are not alone. Many people with a cancer diagnosis do not have the funds available to go through all of the treatment that they wish to. There are, however, various strategies that can aid you with this, such as what follows;

» Fundraising is an option if you are wanting to seek some of the more complex options found in this book.

» Changing your diet and avoiding alcohol.

» Speaking to your local grocery store and explaining your diagnosis or circumstance may lead them to provide you with a wholesale discount on organic produce. (Try to reach out to the company/store owner, as they are the ones that will be more likely to provide a discount or help when or where they can).

» Growing your own vegetables and herbs is an option if you have the space to do so. There are various windowsill herbs that you can grow if space is limited.

» Exercise and mindfulness techniques are free, such as yoga and tai chi.

» Ozone therapy can be done at home with a one-off minimal purchase.

» IV therapies may be discounted to you if you explain your predicament.

» Swapping plastics for glass is a cheap win as you can do this for little or no money if you speak with family, friends, or check out your local charity shops.

» Turn off your WiFi signal to give your cells a break from EMF.

» Use a mix of bicarbonate of soda and water daily to keep your body in an alkalised, and not acidic state.

» Use curcumin and garlic in your foods and as a supplement if you can.

A couple in the USA have podcasts, YouTube videos, and a website called The Stern Method where they openly talk about various fundraising techniques that they used while trying to fund their son's cancer treatment. They have a wealth of advice on this.

If you are not comfortable reaching out to people, you could send an email or ask a family friend to maybe do so on your behalf. You will be amazed at human kindness and compassion at a time like this.

If you are struggling with your finances due to a cancer diagnosis, there are resources available at the Macmillan Cancer Support website for UK residents.

If you are in other parts of the world, please reach out to your local cancer support groups, as there will be local services and offerings available for you to utilise.

****

Chapter Twenty-Seven

How To Prevent Cancer

So we have covered various therapies that are great at fighting cancer, so now we need to cover the various techniques that can be used to help you to prevent it from occurring in the first place.

» **Eat a low GI and predominantly plant-based diet**

This diet allows you to get the most nutrients and avoid the acid and hormones that can be found in dairy and animal products. Try to also avoid simple carbohydrates that create insulin spikes.

» **Try to eat organic when possible**

This allows you to avoid the majority of GMOs, toxins, and pesticides found in foods.

» **Keep a healthy BMI**

Obesity promotes cancer as fat cells secrete transmitters that optimise angiogenesis (the process of which new blood vessels are formed). Angiogenesis plays a huge role in cancer growth, as tumours need a blood supply in order to grow. Tumours can cause angiogenesis by giving off chemical signals that stimulate the process.

» **Exercise daily**

Studies show that even brisk walking for 10 minutes per day will lead to a decreased rate of cancer.

» Turn off the WiFi and other EMF devices when you can

This will allow your body to regenerate and not be bombarded with cell-destroying radiofrequencies 100% of the time.

» Use the cooker and not the microwave

Microwaves nuke your food and kill the bulk of the goodness and nutrients that we should be consuming. You should therefore try to eat your vegetables in a state as close to raw as possible in order to ingest as many nutrients as possible. If heating your food up, it is preferable for you to do this by using the oven and not the microwave.

» Avoid plastics when you can and opt for glass cookware instead

This allows you to stay away from the toxins released from plastic that make their way into your bloodstream.

» Avoid stress or manage it with stress reducing activities, meditation, or deep breathing exercises

Stress indirectly weakens the immune system and the long-term release of hormones relating to stress have been shown to damage DNA and affect the DNA repair process.

» Avoid alcohol

Alcohol is listed as a group 1 carcinogen by The International Agency for Research on Cancer. Alcohol causes a chemical reaction in the body that increases the risk of developing cancer.

» Reduce oxidative stress

This can cause direct damage to the DNA and supress the process of cancer cell death.

» **Avoid dairy**

Dairy has a high level of animal hormones in its produce that, once consumed, can create an imbalance in your body due to the added hormones from this external source.

» **Take your supplements**
» **Make conscious healthy life choices**

****

Chapter Twenty-Eight

Planning For The End

Let's face it, every single one of us has one thing in common and that is the fact that one day we are all going to die. We all just hope and pray that we get as much time as possible on this earth to spend with those that we love and cherish. Whether you are facing a cancer prognosis or not, I would always recommend that your affairs are all in order regardless, so that as and when that fateful day arrives we are organised and can leave knowing that our loved ones are aware of our wishes. The basics that should be covered are listed below:

Hospice Care

Some people assume that a hospice is just the place that you go to die, however, this is not the truth. Hospices provide help, support, and care to anyone that has an incurable illness from the point of diagnosis until the end of their life. You can use a hospice as respite for yourself or to allow your carer to have a break. You can choose to pause the service and take a break if you feel better and then resume the service when you need to. Each hospice would usually have a palliative care team that will work with you or your loved one to ensure that any symptoms are monitored and controlled. You can use the service as an inpatient or as an outpatient, should you choose to use some of the various facilities that may be offered.

Some of the services offered may include:
- » Counselling.
- » Holistic or complimentary therapies, such as acupuncture, massage, or yoga.
- » Rehabilitation.
- » Financial advice.
- » Occupational therapy.

>> Support groups.

>> Bereavement therapy for family and friends.

When initially introduced to a hospice, you should be provided with a leaflet that will allow you to answer questions in relation to your medication and future preferences.

If you are a stage 4 cancer sufferer or under palliative care, there will be questions in relation to your end of life care that may be addressed, such as where you would like your end of life care to take place, whether you would prefer to end your days at home or whether you would prefer to end your days in a hospice or hospital. Any additional decisions in relation to your care can also be addressed, such as any decisions that you may have if you are no longer able to communicate your wishes.

Hospice care in the UK is offered for free as part of the NHS service. If you are in another part of the world, your medical insurance should cover your care. If you do not have medical insurance, there are various charitable organisations that can be approached who should be able to assist you in finding out if there are options available for you for no fee.

Funeral Planning

When forward planning, it may be a good idea to address some of the below questions in relation to yours or your loved one's funeral plans:

>> **What kind of funeral do you want, a burial or cremation?**
   o If a burial, do you have a location requirement?
   o If a cremation, do you have an idea of what you would like to happen to your ashes?
>> **What kind of service would you like, religious or non-religious?**
   o Do you have anyone in particular that you would like to speak at the funeral?
>> **Do you know what kind of casket you would like?**

» Would you like people to carry your coffin and if so who?

» What is your favourite song, or songs that you would like played?

» Do you have any poems that you would like read or prayers said in your service?

» Who would you like to attend the funeral?

» What kind of wake would you like?

» Would you like to have funeral cars?

» Do you have any final resting place wishes or belongings that you would like with you?

Paying For The Funeral

You can contact a local funeral home who will talk you through the funeral planning process and can assist you with creating a funeral plan or package. Your hospice may even provide a service that can help you to make the necessary plans. If you do not want to make the plan but have money set aside for your funeral, let your loved ones know.

There is a leaflet available from Dying Matters called My Funeral Wishes, which you can use to record your final instructions. Alternatively, you can write your wishes down in your last will and testament or in a document that is sometimes called an advanced care plan, which can be found on the internet.

If you do not have funds to pay for your own funeral, your local council or district will arrange the funeral and your loved ones can discuss the offerings with them as and when that time arrives.

There is also help available in the UK from the government by means of The Social Fund that your family may be eligible for if they are in receipt of certain benefits. They would need to visit gov.uk or contact their local benefits office for funeral payment advice.

If you do not want to discuss your own funeral with a loved one as it makes you feel uncomfortable, that's completely OK. However, please bear in mind that if you have certain requests and wants, it may be better to address the subject in order to ensure that your final wishes are adhered to and the people that you have left behind know what you would like for them to do.

****

Chapter Twenty-Nine

Don't Give Up!

Even though the last chapter covered funerals, remember that it is always wise to plan for the inevitable, regardless of our age, health, or circumstance. That chapter was not to dishearten you, but was placed in to ensure that all bases are covered and organised. Cancer has no 'one-size-fits-all' solution, and that is why it is so important to not give up hope, heart, or fight!

If you have the mental and physical ability to keep trying the methods in this book and any other treatments available to you, it may be worth a go as, as stated earlier, that may be the one treatment that interacts with your cells and kick-starts the healing process for you.

We are all different individuals with a different genetic makeup and different ways of working. You or your loved one may be that part of the population that reacts positively to one of the treatments that you are trying.

Remember to take the time to try cellular healing while undertaking these methods, encouraging your cells to interact with the treatment that you are using, and encouraging it to work.

I stumbled upon a prayer that I thought was wonderful from a book called Enriching Our Worship 2. This prayer may provide you with some comfort and strength at this time.

'Comfort Me in Suffering - Loving God, I pray that you will comfort me in my suffering, lend skill to the hands of my healers, and bless the means used for my cure. Give me such confidence in the power of your grace, that even when I am afraid, I may put my whole trust in you; through our Saviour Jesus Christ. Amen. '

Please keep your faith up at this time and remember to learn from your experiences in a positive way as that is what life is about; learning, growing, healing, embracing, and appreciating all that we love and can be thankful for.

May God bless you on your journey. I hope that you have gained insight from this book and I really hope that I have given you some hope that there is a chance that you or your loved one can heal or outlive any prognosis.

****

My Healing Plan

My Healing Plan is an undated planner that I created when I was trying to find ways that could help others that are on a similar journey to my mum.

I created it as a space for people to track where they are now against where they want to be on their journey, healing plan and life.

The space has been designed to allow you to write down details of plans, protocols and treatments that you may wish to try or embark on and is a place where you can journal how you are feeling each day as well as log your to do lists and tasks.

Inside, you will find motivational phrases to keep your positivity up and a space where you can write down what you love and care about as a focus to keep you going and to refer back to. The twelve month planner is in a weekly format and has been left undated so that you can start any time in the year.

My Healing Plan is a safe space that you can use to create your plan to reach health and healing. You can find snippets of advice, guidance, prompts, motivation, and affirmations as well as exercise, nutrition, supplementation, and herb advice that you can include in your mind maps when creating your plans or protocols.

My Healing Plan is available to order from www.ndlondon.co.uk and www.amazon.co.uk.

****

Reference List

Chapter 1:

1. Understanding cancer prognosis, National cancer institute.

Chapter 3:

2. How Chemotherapy drugs work, revised (2019) American Cancer Society.
3. T lymphocytes. Fabbri M, Smart C, Pardi R. T lymphocytes. Int J Biochem Cell Biol. 2003 Jul;35(7):1004-8. doi: 10.1016/ s1357-2725(03)00037-2. PMID: 12672468. https://pubmed.ncbi.nlm.nih.gov/12672468.
4. Immunotherapy. Tendeiro Rego R, Morris EC, Lowdell MW. T-cell receptor gene-modified cells: past promises, present methodologies and future challenges. Cytotherapy. 2019 Mar;21(3):341-357. doi: 10.1016/j.jcyt.2018.12.002. Epub 2019 Jan 14. PMID: 30655164.https://pubmed.ncbi.nlm.nih.gov/30655164/.

Chapter 5 :

1. EMF. Bortkiewicz A. Health effects of Radiofrequency Electromagnetic Fields (RF EMF). *Ind Health.* 2019;57(4):403-405. doi:10.2486/indhealth.57_400.
2. Rife machine. Zimmerman JW, Jimenez H, Pennison MJ, et al. Targeted treatment of cancer with radiofrequency electromagnetic fields amplitude-modulated at tumor-specific frequencies. *Chin J Cancer.* 2013;32(11):573-581. doi:10.5732/cjc.013.10177.

Chapter 6 :

1. PRP. A. M. Elvis and J. S. Ekta, Heliyon. 2020 Mar; 6(3): e03660. 2020 Mar 28. doi: 10.1016/j.heliyon.2020.e03660 PMCID: PMC7113436 , PMID: 32258495.
2. https://www.ncbi.nlm.nih.gov/pmc/articles/PMC7113436/.
3. The biology and function of fibroblasts in cancer. Raghu Kalluri . Nat Rev Cancer. 2016 Aug 23;16(9):582-98. doi: 10.1038/nrc.2016.73.https://pubmed.ncbi.nlm.nih.gov/27550820.
4. The "Yin and Yang" of Platelet-rich Plasma in Breast Reconstruction After Mastectomy or Lumpectomy for Breast Cancer. Spartalis E, Tsilimigras DI, Charalampoudis P, Karachaliou

GS, Moris D, Athanasiou A, Spartalis M, Bolkas V, Dimitroulis D, Nikiteas N. Anticancer Res. 2017 Dec;37(12):6557-6562. doi: 10.21873/anticanres.12112. PMID: 29187430.https://pubmed.ncbi.nlm.nih.gov/29187430/.

Chapter 7:

1. Gerson Therapy. Good thinking society.https://goodthinkingsociety.org/projects/good-thinking-about/good-thinking-about-gerson-therapy/.
2. Gerson Therapy . B Cassileth Oncology (Williston Park). February, 2010. Vol 24, (2):201 , A Molassiotis and others , Integrative Cancer Therapies, March, 2007. Vol 6, (1), 80-88., J Huebner and others. Anticancer Research. 2014 January; 34(1):39-48.
3. https://www.cancerresearchuk.org/about-cancer/cancer-ingeneral/treatment/complementary-alternative-therapies/individual-therapies/gerson.
4. Gerson Therapy. *Extracts from "Trick or Treatment?" by Singh and Ernst, published by Transworld (2008)*.https://goodthinkingsociety.org/projects/good-thinking-about/good-thinking-about-gerson-therapy/.
5. A Cancer Therapy: Results of Fifty Cases by Dr. Gerson, Healing the Gerson Way by Charlotte Gerson , and Liver Detoxification with Coffee Enemas by Morton Walker, DPM excerpted from July 2001 edition of Townsend Newsletter. https://gerson.org/pdfs/How_Coffee_Enemas_Work.pdf.

Chapter 8

1. Vitamin C jabs and cancer (2008), Analysis by Bazian , Edited by NHS Website.
2. https://www.nhs.uk/news/cancer/vitamin-c-jabs-and-cancer/
3. Why high-dose vitamin C kills cancer cells: Low levels of catalase enzyme make cancer cells vulnerable to high-dose vitamin C. University of Iowa Health Care.ScienceDaily, 9 January 2017. <www.sciencedaily.com/releases/2017/01/170109134014.htm.
4. Synergistic effect of fasting-mimicking diet and vitamin C against *KRAS* mutated cancers .Di Tano, M., Raucci, F., Vernieri, C. *et al.Nat Commun* 11, 2332 (2020). https://doi.org/10.1038/s41467-20-16243-3.
5. A combo of fasting plus vitamin C is effective for hard-to-treat cancers . University of Southern California (2020).

https://www.eurekalert.org/pub_releases/2020-05/uosc-aco051220.php.
6. High doses of vitamin C to improve cancer treatment passes human safety trial. Science Daily. (2017, March 30).. Retrieved September 29, 2020 from www.sciencedaily.com/releases/2017/03/170330142341.htm.

Chapter 9:

1. Ozone therapy: A clinical review. J Nat Sci Biol Med. 2011 Jan-Jun; 2(1): 66–70. , doi: 10.4103/0976-9668.82319 , PMCID: PMC3312702 , PMID: 22470237.
2. https://www.ncbi.nlm.nih.gov/pmc/articles/PMC3312702/.
3. Ozone Therapy as Adjuvant for Cancer Treatment: Is Further Research Warranted. A. M. Elvis and J. S. Ekta , Evid Based Complement Alternat Med. 2018; 2018: 7931849. , Published online 2018 Sep 9. doi: 10.1155/2018/7931849 , PMCID: PMC6151231 , PMID: 30271455 https://www.ncbi.nlm.nih.gov/pmc/articles/PMC6151231/.
4. Dichloroacetate (DCA) and Cancer: An Overview towards Clinical Applications",Tiziana Tataranni, Claudia Piccoli Oxidative Medicine and Cellular Longevity, vol. 2019, Article ID 8201079, 14 pages, 2019. https://doi.org/10.1155/2019/8201079.
5. https://www.hindawi.com/journals/omcl/2019/8201079/.

Chapter 10:

1. Hydrogen Peroxide . Medically reviewed by Yamini Ranchod, Ph.D., M.S. — Written by Jacquelyn Cafasso — Updated on August 28, 2020 https://www.healthline.com/health/hydrogen-peroxide-cancer.
2. Hydrogen peroxide fuels aging, inflammation, cancer metabolism and metastasis: the seed and soil also needs "fertilizer".Lisanti MP, Martinez-Outschoorn UE, Lin Z, et al. Cell Cycle. 2011;10(15):2440-2449. doi:10.4161/cc.10.15.16870.
3. https://www.ncbi.nlm.nih.gov/pmc/articles/PMC3180186/
4. DCA. Medicor Cancer Clinic , Dr. Akbur Kahn, https://medicorcancer.com/medical-director/.

Chapter 12

1. Hyperthermia in Cancer Treatment_ as published by the National Cancer Institute.

https://www.cancer.gov/about-cancer/treatment/types/surgery/hyperthermia-fact-sheet#:~:text=Hyperthermia%20(also%20called%20thermal%20therapy,to%20normal%20tissues%20(1).

Chapter 14:

1. How to Reduce Cancer-Causing Toxins in Your Home. Patient Empowerment Network.
2. https://powerfulpatients.org/2018/05/25/how-to-reduce-cancer-causing-toxins-in-your-home/.
3. The best chemical-free makeup tried and tested by beauty editors. Winter .L (2019) Glamour magazinehttps://www.glamourmagazine.co.uk/gallery/the-best-chemical-free-makeup-tried-and-tested.

Chapter 15:

1. Intermittent Fasting and Cancer Andrea S. Blevins Primeau, (2018) https://www.cancertherapyadvisor.com/home/tools/fact-sheets/intermittent-fasting-and-cancer/.
2. The Roles of Autophagy in Cancer. Yun CW, Lee SH. *Int J Mol Sci*. 2018;19(11):3466. Published 2018 Nov 5. doi:10.3390/ijms19113466. https://www.ncbi.nlm.nih.gov/pmc/articles/PMC6274804/#:~:text=In%20cancer%20cells%2C%20autophagy%20suppresses,by%20a%20series%20of%20proteins.

Chapter 16:

1. Five Popular Diets: Are they right for cancer survivors?. https://www.rogelcancercenter.org/living-with-cancer/nutrition/five-popular-diets-are-they-right-cancer-survivors. Fall, 2019 issue of Thrive.
2. Dr Sebi diet. www.drsebicellfood.com.

Chapter 19:

1. Wikihow, how to make rick Simpson oil (2020). https://www.wikihow.com/Make-Rick-Simpson-Oil.

Chapter 20:

1. Repurposed drugs for cancer . www.careoncologyclinic.com/The Care Oncology Clinic in Harley street, London.
2. Redo Org, list of repurposed drugs , www.redo-project.org/.

Chapter 21:

1. Biosept test, RGCC test & Navarro HCG test. https://biocept.com , http://www.rgcc-group.com , https://www.navarromedicalclinic.com.

Chapter 23:

1. Bioscan. Integrative Wellness Group. https://integrativewellnessgroup.com/service/allergy-testing-bioscan-srt.
2. Releasing emotional turbulence, Deepak Chopra.
3. https://www.gaiam.com/blogs/discover/deepak-chopras-7-step-exercise-to-release-emotional-turbulence.
4. Meditation. Cancer research UK. https://www.cancerresearchuk.org/about-cancer/cancer-ingeneral/treatment/complementary-alternative-therapies/individual-therapies/meditation.
5. Meditation . N.D. London , Anxious about being Anxious, simple techniques to calm the mind www.ndlondon.co.uk.

Chapter 24:

1. Exercise . Science Nordic website.https://sciencenordic.com/cancer-denmark-fitness/how-exercise-can-slow-the-spread-of-cancer/1450630.

Chapter 25:

1. Clinical trials Cancer.gov website. https://www.cancer.gov/about-cancer/treatment/clinical-trials/search.
2. SapC-DOPS . University of Cincinnati, Research points to potential new treatment for pancreatic cancer (2020) . https://medicalxpress.com/news/2020-06-potential-treatment-pancreatic-cancer.html.

Chapter 26:

1. Make money one less worry. Macmillan Cancer Support. https://www.macmillan.org.uk/get-involved/campaigns/money-worries#275622.
2. My Funeral Wishes. Dying Matters. https://www.dyingmatters.org/sites/default/files/files/My%20Funeral%20Wishes%202017.pdf.
3. The Social Fund. www.Gov.co.uk.

Treatment centres and tests:

1. www.fayecoulson.com/Biomagnetism therapy, UK London.
2. www.aurorscalartechnology.com/en/naturopathy-therapy/ - Eindhoven Rife therapy, Netherlands.
3. www.balancedhealthclinic.co.uk/ - Balanced health clinic –Isle of Man UK.
4. www.bodyvibrant.co.uk/ - Colonic hydrotherapy, rectal ozone , Berkshire , UK.
5. www.drrowendrsu.com/about/- Dr Robert Rowan & Dr Terri Su Innovative Biologic clinic in Santa Barbara CA.
6. www.drbuttar.com/ - The Centre for advanced medicine and clinical research , USA.
7. www.medicorcancer.com/- Medicor cancer centre, CA.
8. www.hoxseybiomedical.com/- Hoxey Clinic, Mexico.
9. www.oasisofhope.com/- Oasis of Hope clinic , Mexico.
10. https://hope4cancer.com , Hope For Cancer Clinic, Cancun, Mexico.

Resources

1. The Truth about cancer a global quest –Docuseries https://go2.thetruthaboutcancer.com/agq-encore/own/?p=silver.
2. The Cancer Directory by Dr. Rosy Daniel.

RGCC test results

I have decided to make my mother's RGCC test results for natural substances available for information purposes only. By seeing these test results, you may feel that the test could be beneficial for yourself or your loved one. The results show the percentage that certain natural substances work towards killing individual cancer cells for your specific gene type and the results are based off your blood sample analysis.

 R.G.C.C. - RESEARCH GENETIC CANCER CENTRE S.A.

Dear Colleague,

We send you the results from the analysis on a patient ..... suffering from non small cell lung carcinoma stage IV. The sample that was sent to us for analysis was a sample of 20ml of whole blood that contained EDTA-Ca as anti-coagulant, and packed with an ice pack.

In our laboratory we made the following:

- We isolated the malignant cells using Oncoquick with a membrane that isolates malignant cells from normal cells. Then we centrifuged at 350g for 10 min and we collected the supernatant with the malignant cells. Then we proceed to isolation of malignant cells from mononuclear cells by negative selection.
- Then we developed forty six cell cultures in a fetal calf serum media. In each culture of the well plate we added a biological modifier substance [wie Quercetin, Super Artemisinin, Poly- MVA, C-statin, Ascorbic acid, Ukrain, Bio D Mulsion NuMedica Micellized D3, Aromat8-PN, Theaflavin, Salicinium, Fucoidan, Breastin, Onkobel Pro, GcMAF (Big Harmony), Polyphenole CA, Mito Booster, Mitochondrien Formular Artesunate, Doxycycline, Apigenin, Angiostop, Agaricus Blazei Murill, Butyric Acid, Pure Quercetin, Alpha lipoic Acid, Ribraxx, CoQ10, Curcumin (turmeric), Vitanox, Mistletoe, Amygdalin-(B17), Thymex, Salvestrol, Virxcan, Avemar pulvis, Boswellia Serratta, Cordyceps Sinensis, Oxaloacetate (Cronaxal), Lycopene, Paw-Paw, Indol 3 Carbinol, Melatonin, Naltrexone, Resveratrol, DCA (dichloroacetate), Genistein, DDG, Artecin, VascuStatin, Frankincense, GcMAF (Big Harmony III), Polyphenole CA III, Mito booster II] that is used in clinical application. Then we developed those cultures and we harvested a sample every 24 hours and made the following assays:
- In the culture that contains all the substances we measure the apoptotic ability using the oncogen apoptosis kit.
- In the culture that contains the ukrain we measure the inhibition of tyrosine kinase catalytic ability from the growth factor receptors (EGF-r, IGF-r) and the production of cytokines PMBC
- In the culture that contains quercetinwe measure theinhibition of EGF and IGF.
- In the culture that contains indol-3-carbinol we measure the inhibition of VEGF and FGF and PDGF.
- In the culture that contains the mistletoe we measure the inhibition of tyrosine kinase catalytic ability from the growth factor receptors (EGF-r, IGF-r) and the production of cytokines and the increase of PMBC.
- In the culture that contains the ascorbic acid we measure the catalytic activity of GSH and GSSG (redox reaction) and the induction of cytochrome C (apoptosis).
- In the culture that contains the PolyMVA we measure the catalytic activity of GSH and GSSG (redox reaction) and the induction of cytochrome C (apoptosis).
- In the culture that contains the super artemisinin we measure the catalytic activity of GSH and GSSG (redox reaction for free radical sincesuper artemisinin binds free radicals with the iron molecule), the inhibition of VEGF, FGF and PDGF (since it acts to the angiogenesis cascade reactions) and the induction of cytochrome C (apoptosis).

Class I (cytotoxic Agents)

Activation of Caspace (especially 3 and 9) and cytochrom C re

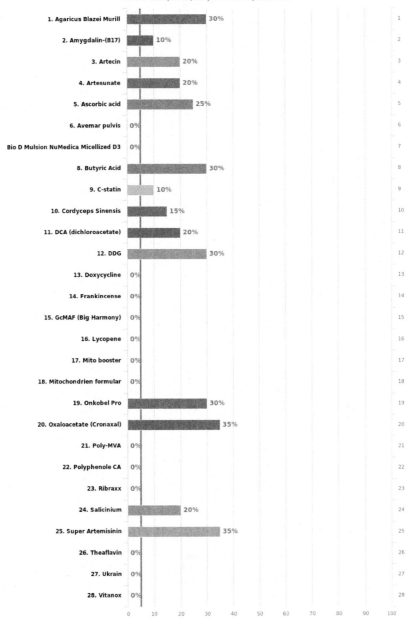

1. Agaricus Blazei Murill	30%
2. Amygdalin-(B17)	10%
3. Artecin	20%
4. Artesunate	20%
5. Ascorbic acid	25%
6. Avemar pulvis	0%
Bio D Mulsion NuMedica Micellized D3	0%
8. Butyric Acid	30%
9. C-statin	10%
10. Cordyceps Sinensis	15%
11. DCA (dichloroacetate)	20%
12. DDG	30%
13. Doxycycline	0%
14. Frankincense	0%
15. GcMAF (Big Harmony)	0%
16. Lycopene	0%
17. Mito booster	0%
18. Mitochondrien formular	0%
19. Onkobel Pro	30%
20. Oxaloacetate (Cronaxal)	35%
21. Poly-MVA	0%
22. Polyphenole CA	0%
23. Ribraxx	0%
24. Salicinium	20%
25. Super Artemisinin	35%
26. Theaflavin	0%
27. Ukrain	0%
28. Vitanox	0%

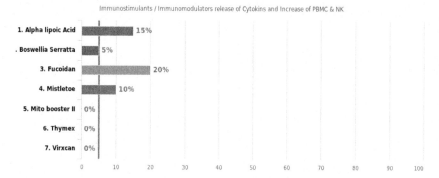

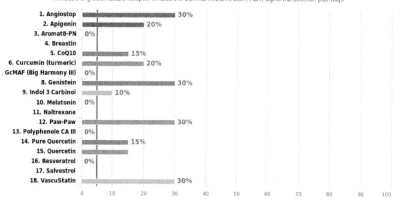

CONCLUSION: *It seems that this specific population of malignant cell have greater sensitivity in Agaricus Blazei Murill, in Amygdalin-(B17), in Artecin, in Artesunate, in Ascorbic acid, in Butyric Acid, in C-statin, in Cordyceps Sinensis, in DCA (dichloroacetate), in DDG, in Onkobel Pro, in Oxaloacetate (Cronaxal), in Salicinium, in Super Artemisinin, in Alpha lipoic Acid, in Fucoidan, in Mistletoe, in Angiostop, in Apigenin, in CoQ10, in Curcumin (turmeric), in Genistein, in Indol 3 Carbinol, in Paw-Paw, in Pure Quercetin, in Quercetin, in VascuStatin and less in Avemar pulvis, in Bio D Mulsion NuMedica Micellized D3, in Doxycycline, in Frankincense, in GcMAF (Big Harmony), in Lycopene, in Mito booster, in Mitochondrien formular, in Poly-MVA, in Polyphenole CA, in Ribraxx, in Theaflavin, in Ukrain, in Vitanox, in Boswellia Serratta, in Mito booster II, in*

142

Thymex, in Virxcan, in Aromat8-PN, in Breastin, in GcMAF (Big Harmony III), in Melatonin, in Naltrexone, in Polyphenole CA III, in Resveratrol, in Salvestrol.

This study is known as an Ex-Vivo type study (testing the actual tumour stem cells of an individual outside their body). This test will tell us what natural substances will induce apoptosis via the cytochrome c (esp. caspase 3 & 9 pathways) after the tumour stem cells and a single product have been in contact, in a well plate for 48 hours. We have found this test to be very accurate over the past 10+ years and thousands of test. However, it cannot take into account the many combinations of natural substances or the physiological dynamics of each individual that are required for life. We are also aware that natural substances can have a wide variety of additional benefits that may assist healthy individuals, as well as those with cancer. Therefore, even if a product shows not to induce apoptosis, on this test, it most likely will have many other benefits especially when used in combination with other therapies your health care provider may use. This is when you must rely on the skill, knowledge and training of your health care provider and their years of clinical experience (successes and failures) with the many various combinations which they have found to work in a clinical setting. The body is a wonderful, magnificent, dynamic organism and very complex.

Should you wish to undertake any personalised testing, it is recommended that you do your research to ensure that it is the best way for you or your loved one to move forward. My mum's complete RGCC test results can be found at www.ndlondon.co.uk.

****

Check Out
My Other Books

Thank you so much for taking the time to read my book.

Please visit www.ndlondon.co.uk
to join my mailing list and to check out my other books.

Affirmations: 33 affirmations that will transform your life.
How to manifest all that you want, wish, and desire.

Anxious about being anxious:
Simple techniques to calm the mind.

My Healing Plan:
The ultimate journal to help you to embark on your healing journey.

If you have felt that this book has helped you in any way please leave a review on Amazon, as your reviews are greatly appreciated.

www.ndlondon.co.uk
www.divine-distribution.co.uk

Printed in Great Britain
by Amazon

Printed in Great Britain
by Amazon